IMMEDIATE LIFE SUPPORT FOR DENTISTS

A Step-By-Step Guide

By

Blessing Isaackson

Disclaimer

This handbook is for **learning and training purposes only**.

- It explains the principles of Immediate Life Support for Dentists.
- It does **not replace professional training or certification**.
- Always follow local guidelines and ensure you have the proper skills before applying these steps.
- The author and publisher are not liable for misuse of the information.

Second Edition

ISBN: 978-1-0683557-2-1

Contents

Foreword

Dental professionals are often the first responders when a medical emergency arises within the practice. In those critical moments, confidence, clarity, and prompt action can make the difference between life and death. *Immediate Life Support for Dentists: A Step-by-Step Guide* has been developed by **Fairview Training Ltd** to equip every member of the dental team with the essential knowledge and practical skills required to recognise, respond to, and manage medical emergencies calmly and effectively.

At Fairview Training Ltd, we understand that effective education must be clear, practical, and accessible. Learners gain the greatest benefit from structured guidance, visual clarity, and explanations that translate clinical guidance into real-world application. This handbook has been written with that educational philosophy at its core.

The content reflects current guidance from the **Resuscitation Council UK** and **NICE**, as well as best practice from emergency care and dental settings. Each section is designed to support both initial learning and rapid reference in practice. Whether used by students, newly qualified clinicians, or experienced practitioners refreshing their skills, this guide aims to strengthen understanding and enhance emergency preparedness.

Our aim is to empower dental teams to act decisively, safely, and effectively when it matters most. Every patient deserves a team that is prepared. Every clinician deserves training that builds confidence. And every dental practice deserves a culture in which emergency readiness is not optional, but fundamental.

We thank you for your ongoing commitment to patient safety and continuous professional development. It is our privilege at **Fairview Training Ltd** to support you in maintaining the highest standards of care.

Fairview Training Ltd
Education & Clinical Training Team

Glossary of Key Terms

Abdominal Thrusts

A first-aid technique used to relieve severe airway obstruction in a choking adult or child by applying inward–upward pressure below the ribcage.

Adrenal Insufficiency

A condition where the adrenal glands fail to produce adequate cortisol, potentially leading to collapse during stress or illness.

AED (Automated External Defibrillator)

A portable device that analyses heart rhythm and delivers a shock if needed to treat life-threatening arrhythmias such as VF or pulseless VT.

Airway

The passage through which air enters and leaves the lungs. Must be kept open during emergencies using techniques such as head-tilt, chin-lift.

Anaphylaxis

A severe, life-threatening allergic reaction causing airway swelling, breathing difficulty, and circulatory collapse.

Asystole

A cardiac arrest rhythm showing no electrical activity — a flat line on the ECG. Not shockable.

AVPU

A rapid assessment tool for consciousness: Alert, Voice responsive, Pain responsive, Unresponsive.

Immediate Life Support (BLS)

A set of emergency procedures including airway management, rescue breaths, and chest compressions to maintain life until advanced help arrives.

Blood Pressure (BP)

The force of blood against artery walls is recorded as systolic over diastolic (e.g., 120/80 mmHg).

Brachial Pulse

Pulse felt on the inner upper arm, commonly used in infants.

Buccal Midazolam

A fast-acting benzodiazepine administered inside the cheek to stop prolonged seizures.

Capillary Refill Time (CRT)

A quick test of circulation; normal refill is under 2 seconds.

Cardiac Arrest

A sudden loss of heart function, breathing, and consciousness requiring immediate CPR and defibrillation.

Carotid Pulse

Pulse felt on either side of the neck; used in adult cardiac arrest assessment.

Chain of Survival

A sequence of actions that improve survival from cardiac arrest: early recognition, early CPR, early defibrillation, and post-resuscitation care.

Chest Compressions

Rhythmic pressing on the chest to circulate blood during CPR.

Choking (Mild/Severe)

Airway obstruction caused by a foreign body. Severe choking requires abdominal or chest thrusts.

Consent

Permission for treatment given voluntarily, with capacity, and after receiving adequate information.

Convulsive Status Epilepticus

A seizure lasting more than 5 minutes or repeated seizures without recovery is a medical emergency.

CPR (Cardiopulmonary Resuscitation)

A lifesaving technique combining chest compressions and rescue breaths to maintain circulation and oxygenation.

Defibrillation

Delivery of an electric shock to restore a normal heart rhythm in shockable cardiac arrest rhythms.

DNACPR / DNAR

A documented decision not to attempt CPR if the patient arrests. Does not limit other treatments.

DRABCDE

Primary survey sequence: Danger, Response, Airway, Breathing, Circulation, Disability, Exposure.

Epilepsy

A neurological condition characterised by recurrent unprovoked seizures.

Face Shield

A barrier device used during rescue breaths to reduce infection risk.

Focal Seizure

A seizure originating in one part of the brain, sometimes progressing to generalised activity.

Gillick Competence

A legal principle allowing children under 16 to consent to treatment if they demonstrate sufficient understanding.

Heat Exhaustion

A heat-related illness with elevated body temperature (up to 40°C), sweating, dizziness, and weakness.

Heat Stroke

A life-threatening condition where core temperature exceeds 40°C, causing confusion, collapse, or seizures.

Hydrocortisone

A corticosteroid used in severe asthma or adrenal crisis to reduce inflammation.

Hypotension

Low blood pressure, typically systolic <90 mmHg.

Hypothermia

Abnormally low body temperature below 35°C.

Ipratropium Bromide

An anticholinergic bronchodilator used alongside salbutamol in severe asthma attacks.

Jaw Thrust

An airway-opening technique used when trauma is suspected.

LLF (Look, Listen, Feel)

A method for assessing breathing by observing chest movement, listening for breath sounds, and feeling airflow.

Nebuliser

A device that converts liquid medication into a mist for inhalation.

Oxygen Saturation (SpO_2)

Percentage of oxygen-bound haemoglobin measured using a pulse oximeter.

Pocket Mask

A device used to deliver rescue breaths with a one-way valve.

Prednisolone

An oral corticosteroid used in moderate to severe asthma exacerbations.

Primary Survey

A rapid assessment to identify and treat life-threatening conditions using DRABCDE.

Pulse Oximeter

A non-invasive device that measures oxygen saturation and pulse rate.

Radial Pulse

Pulse felt on the thumb side of the wrist; commonly used in conscious adults.

Recovery Position

A safe side-lying position is used for unconscious but breathing patients to maintain airway patency.

Rescue Breaths

Breaths delivered during CPR provide oxygen to the lungs.

Salbutamol

A fast-acting bronchodilator used to relieve acute asthma symptoms.

Seizure

A sudden burst of abnormal electrical activity in the brain causes involuntary movements or altered awareness.

Shock (Circulatory)

A life-threatening condition where tissues receive inadequate blood flow.

Sinoatrial (SA) Node

The heart's natural pacemaker that initiates electrical impulses.

Spacer

A chamber used with inhalers to improve medication delivery to the lungs.

Status Epilepticus

A prolonged seizure requiring urgent medical treatment.

Stroke

A sudden interruption of the blood supply to the brain causes neurological deficits.

Tachycardia

A fast heart rate, typically over 100 beats per minute.

Terbutaline

A bronchodilator used as an alternative to salbutamol in asthma management.

Tonic–Clonic Seizure

A generalised seizure involving stiffening (tonic) followed by rhythmic jerking (clonic) movements.

Ventilation

Movement of air in and out of the lungs; may be assisted during CPR.

Ventricular Fibrillation (VF)

A chaotic, life-threatening heart rhythm requiring immediate defibrillation.

Ventricular Tachycardia (VT)

A fast, abnormal rhythm from the ventricles; pulseless VT is a shockable cardiac arrest rhythm.

Aims of Immediate Life Support

In line with Resuscitation Council UK (2025) and NICE guidance, Immediate Life Support aims to:

- **Preserve life** — respond rapidly and effectively to prevent avoidable death.
- **Prevent deterioration** — identify early warning signs and intervene before the patient's condition worsens.
- **Promote recovery** — provide timely support and stabilisation until advanced medical help takes over.

Infection Control

START: PATIENT ARRIVES

↓

1. HAND HYGIENE
• Wash or sanitise hands
• Remove jewellery

↓

2. PPE SELECTION
• Gloves
• Mask/respirator
• Eye protection
• Apron/gown

↓

3. PREPARE OPERATORY

- Disinfect surfaces
- Set up clean tray
- Check ventilation

↓

4. DURING PROCEDURE

- Use high-volume suction
- Avoid aerosol spread
- Maintain aseptic field

↓

5. SHARPS SAFETY

- Do not recap needles
- Dispose immediately
- Use approved sharps bin

↓

6. INSTRUMENT PROCESSING

- Clean → Inspect → Pack
- Sterilise (HTM 01-05)
- Store aseptically

↓

7. ENVIRONMENT CLEANING

- Wipe all surfaces
- Disinfect chair & HVE
- Replace barriers

↓

8. WASTE DISPOSAL

- Segregate correctly
- Seal clinical waste
- Remove PPE safely

↓

9. FINAL HAND HYGIENE

- Wash or sanitise hands
- Document if required

↓

END

Communication, SBAR & Consent in Dental Practice

1. Why Communication Matters in Dentistry

Effective communication:

Keeps patients **safe**

- Builds **trust**
- Reduces complaints and errors
- Is a **GDC requirement** (Standards for the Dental Team)

Communication in dentistry happens:

- With **patients**
- Between **team members**
- With **external services** (e.g. 999, GDPs, hospitals)

2. Patient Communication: The Basics

Use Clear, Simple Language

- Avoid jargon
- Explain procedures step-by-step
- Check understanding ("Can you tell me what you've understood?")

Be Patient-Centred

- Listen actively
- Acknowledge fears or concerns
- Adapt communication for anxiety, disability, or language needs

Remember: Communication is two-way, not just giving information.

3. SBAR: Structured Clinical Communication

SBAR is a structured way to communicate valuable information clearly and safely.

What SBAR Stands For

Letter	Meaning	What to Say
S	Situation	What is happening now?
B	Background	Relevant medical/dental history
A	Assessment	What you think is wrong
R	Recommendation	What you need to happen next

SBAR Example (Dental Emergency)

S – Situation
"This is a dental practice. I have a patient with suspected anaphylaxis."

B – Background
"They had local anaesthetic and developed wheeze and hypotension."

A – Assessment
"They are conscious but struggling to breathe."

R – Recommendation
"We need an emergency ambulance urgently."

SBAR is especially useful when:

- Calling **999**
- Handing over to paramedics
- Escalating concerns within the team

4. Consent in Dental Practice

What Is Consent?

Consent is the patient's **permission** for treatment, given:

- **Voluntarily**
- With **capacity**
- After receiving **enough information**

Types of Consent

- **Implied** – e.g. opening mouth for examination
- **Verbal** – spoken agreement (most routine dental care)
- **Written** – for complex or invasive procedures

5. Valid Consent: The 3 Key Elements

1. Capacity

- Patient can understand, retain, weigh information, and communicate a decision
- Adults are assumed to have capacity unless proven otherwise

2. Information

Explain:

- What the procedure is
- Benefits and risks
- Alternatives (including no treatment)
- Costs (where relevant)

3. Voluntariness

- No pressure or coercion
- Patient can change their mind at any time

Consent is a process, not a form.

6. Consent in Special Situations

Children & Young People

- **Gillick competence** may apply
- Otherwise, consent from someone with **parental responsibility**

Medical Emergencies

- If the patient lacks capacity and delay risks life:

    - Treat in the **patient's best interests**
    - Document clearly

7. Documentation & Record Keeping

Always record:

- What was explained
- Questions asked by the patient
- Consent given (and how)
- Any refusal or withdrawal of consent

Good records = good protection for patients and staff.

DNACPR (Do Not Attempt CPR) in a Dental Practice

- A **DNACPR decision** is a **clinically recorded instruction** stating that **CPR should not be attempted** if a patient suffers a cardiac arrest in the dental setting.
- It **applies only to CPR** and **does not limit any other dental or medical care**, including oxygen, airway support, pain relief, or comfort measures.
- Respecting DNACPR decisions in a dental emergency:
    - Ensures the patient's **wishes and best interests** are followed
    - Maintains **dignity and comfort**
    - Avoids **futile or potentially harmful interventions**
- Dental teams should:
    - **Check for a DNACPR order** during patient assessment if relevant
    - **Call 999** and provide full handover, noting the DNACPR status
    - **Continue all other emergency care** as appropriate

PRIMARY SURVEY – DRABCDE

Rapid assessment to identify and treat life-threatening problems

D – DANGER

✓ Check the area is safe

✓ Protect yourself, the patient, and others

→ **Do not put yourself at risk**

R – RESPONSE

✓ Talk to the patient

✓ Gently shake shoulders

✓ Ask simple questions

→ **No response = shout for help**

A – AIRWAY

✓ Is the airway open and clear?

✓ Look for obstruction (vomit, swelling, foreign body)

✓ Open airway (head-tilt chin-lift / jaw thrust if trauma)

→ **A blocked airway kills first**

B – BREATHING

✓ Look, listen, feel for breathing

✓ Assess rate, depth, effort

✓ Give high-flow oxygen if available

→ **Not breathing normally = start CPR**

C – CIRCULATION

✓ Check pulse and skin colour

✓ Control severe bleeding

✓ Look for signs of shock

→ **Treat life-threatening bleeding immediately**

D – DISABILITY

✓ Assess consciousness (AVPU)

✓ Check blood glucose if indicated

✓ Look for seizure or stroke signs

→ **Sudden changes are serious**

E – EXPOSURE

✓ Look for rashes, swelling, and injuries

✓ Check for medical alert jewellery

✓ Maintain dignity and keep warm

→ **Exposure gives vital clues**

KEY REMINDERS

✓ Treat problems **as you find them**

✓ Work **top to bottom**

✓ **Repeat DRABCDE** if the patient deteriorates

✓ Call for help early

Chain of Survival

The **2025 Resuscitation Council UK chain of survival** highlights:

Absolutely — here is a version that **matches the four-link structure and wording style shown in your image**, while still staying aligned with current RCUK guidance.

CHAIN OF SURVIVAL

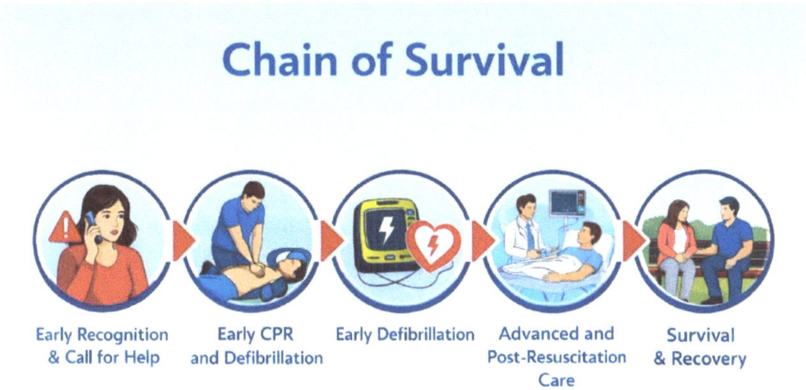

1. Early Recognition & Call for Help

Identify cardiac arrest quickly by checking responsiveness and breathing. Activate emergency services immediately so the right help is on the way.

2. Early CPR and Defibrillation

Start high-quality chest compressions without delay and use an AED as soon as it becomes available. These two actions together give the best chance of restoring a shockable rhythm.

3. Advanced and Post-Resuscitation Care

Once professionals arrive, they provide advanced life support, treat reversible causes, stabilise the patient, and deliver structured post-ROSC care in the hospital.

4. Survival & Recovery

Ongoing hospital treatment, rehabilitation, and psychological support help the patient recover and return to daily life.

Calling for Help

When calling 999/112 (or 2222 in NHS hospitals), provide:

- Your exact location.
- The type of help required.
- Patient's name and number of casualties.
- Clear description of the situation.

Assessing Vital Signs

Airway: Ensure no obstruction.
Breathing: Normal rate = 12–20 breaths/min. Oxygen saturation should be **94–98% (SpO_2).**
Circulation:

- **Pulse:** Check radial, carotid, or brachial pulse.
- **Blood pressure:** Normal adult BP ≈ 120/80 mmHg.
- **Capillary refill:** <2 seconds is normal.
  Temperature:
- Normal: 36–37°C.
- Mild hypothermia: 32–35°C.
- Severe heat illness: >40°C (heat stroke).

Temperature

Digital Thermometer—This is the most accurate thermometer. It can take the temperature orally, in the armpit, or rectally.

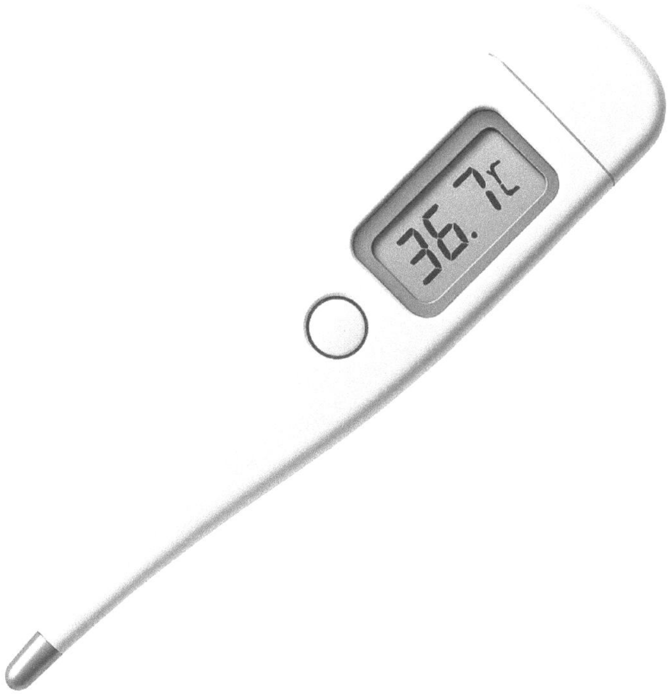

Tympanic Thermometer: is a thermometer that measures the temperature inside the patient's ears by measuring the infrared heat inside the ear.

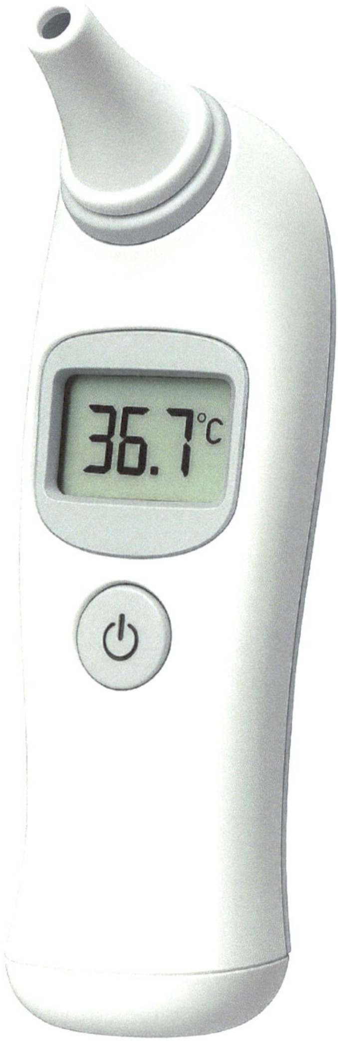

Temporal Thermometer-forehead thermometer. They are not as dependable as digital thermometers. They are placed or pointed at the forehead. They measure the infrared heat generated by the forehead.

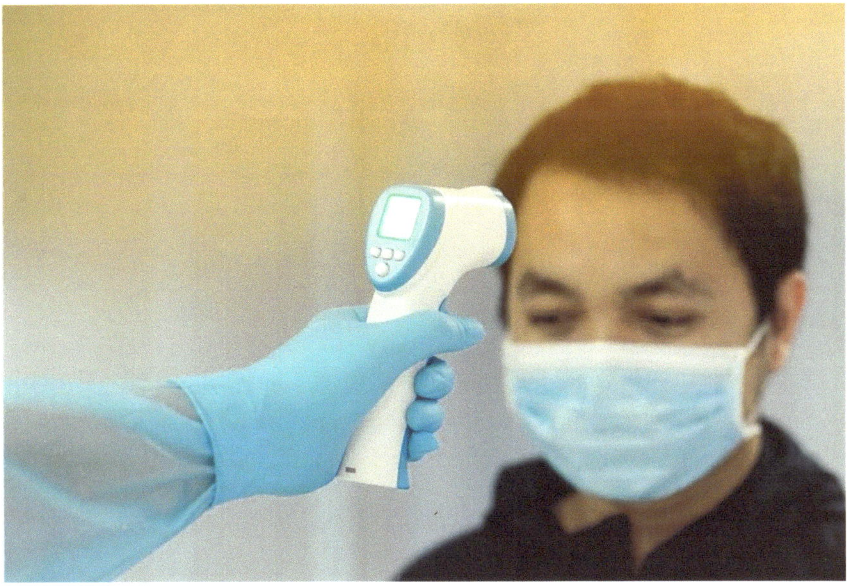

Normal human temperature: between 36° C and 37° C and maintained in the range of 35.8°C- 38.2°C.

Mild Hypothermia– 32-35°C

Moderate Hypothermia– 28-32°C

Severe Hypothermia– less than 28°C

Heat Stress- a mild form of heat-related illness.

Heat Exhaustion is a more severe form of heat-related illness in which the core body temperature is between 37°C and 40°C.

Heat Stroke: core body temperature of over 40°C.

Pulse

This is the number of times the heart beats over a given period, usually a minute.

Pulse locations.

- **Carotid- this** can be taken on either side of the neck. **Brachial, between** the biceps and the triceps, Femoral, upper thigh, near the groin
- **Radial**- radial artery between the wrist bone and the tendon on the thumb side of the wrist.
- **Popliteal** is in the back of the knee
- **Posterior Tibial**- the area behind the medial malleolus.
- The dorsal is in the middle section of the dorsal part of the foot near the ankle.
- **Radial Pulse: radial** artery between the wrist bone and the tendon on the thumb side of the wrist and the inner part of the forearm.

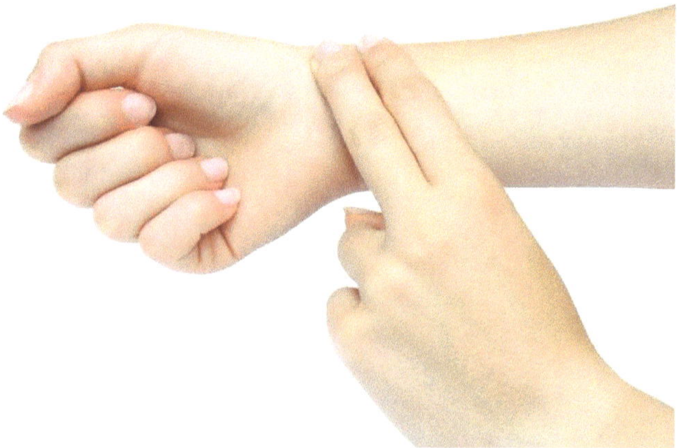

Carotid pulse

- Carotid-this can be taken on either side of the neck.

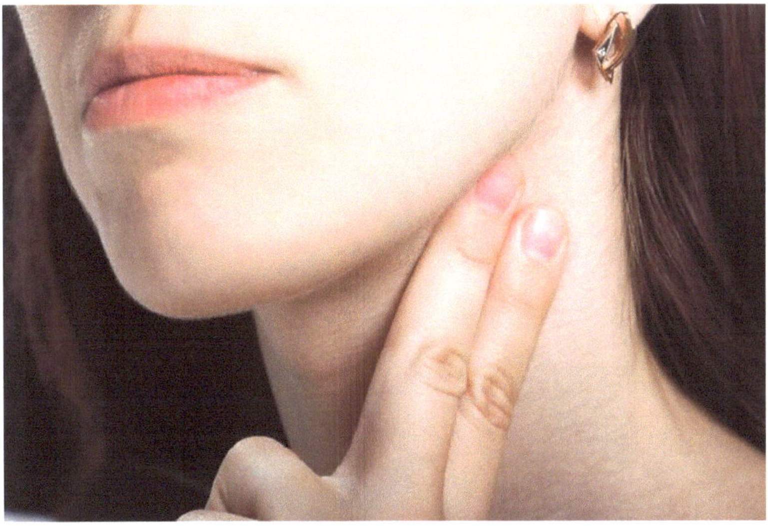

BRACHIAL PULSE

This is located between the biceps and the triceps.

Checking the **brachial pulse**:

- Position the arm slightly bent with the palm facing up.
- Place your **index and middle fingers** on the **inner upper arm**, just above the elbow crease.
- Press gently until you feel the pulse.

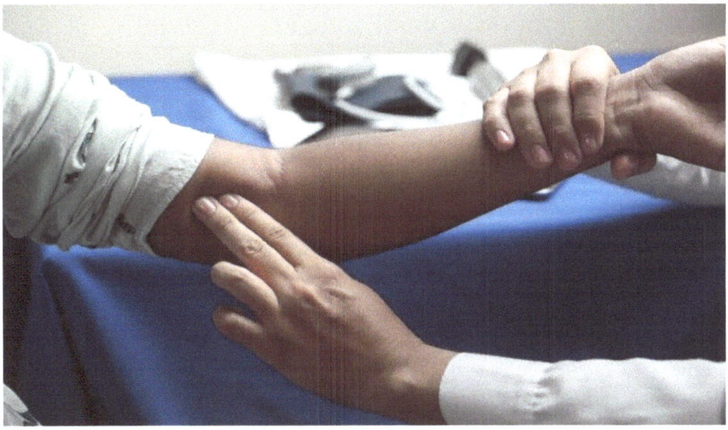

Pulse Oximeter

A **pulse oximeter** is a small, non-invasive device that clips onto a fingertip to measure your blood's oxygen saturation (SpO_2) and pulse rate using light sensor.

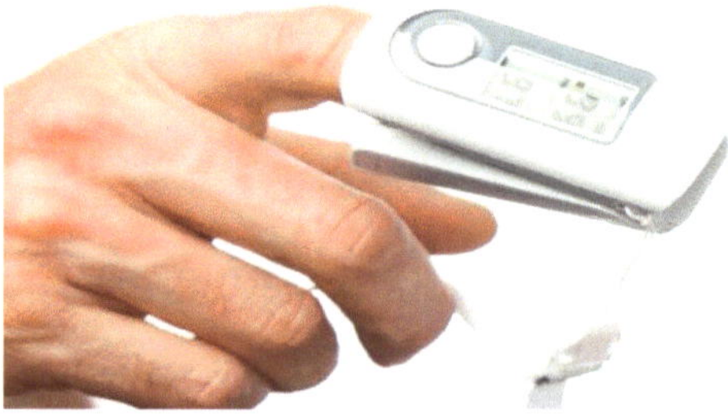

A **pulse oximeter** has **no absolute contraindications**, but it may be **unreliable or inappropriate** in certain situations:

- **Poor peripheral perfusion** (e.g. shock, hypothermia)
- **Movement or tremors**
- **Nail polish, acrylic nails, or henna**
- **Carbon monoxide poisoning** (false normal readings)
- **Severe anaemia**
- **Skin pigmentation or ambient light interference**
- **Incorrect probe placement or damaged sensors**

It should always be used alongside **clinical assessment**, not as a standalone diagnostic tool.

BLOOD PRESSURE

This measures blood pressure within blood vessels. The blood pressure record has two measurements: Systolic blood Pressure is the BP when the ventricles contract and blood is forced off the heart. This is the higher reading of the BP.

Diastolic Blood Pressure is the BP when the ventricles relax. This is the lower reading of the blood pressure.

Blood pressure is measured in millimetres of mercury (mmHg) and is usually recorded as systolic over diastolic—120/80.

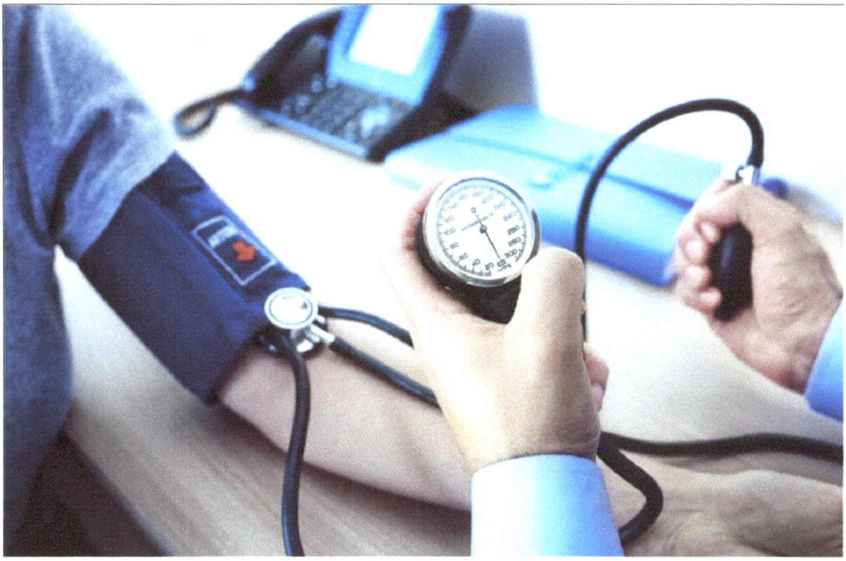

Blood Pressure Values

Normal Range

- Systolic -120-129 mmHg
- Diastolic-80-84 mmHg

Hypertension Systolic 140 or higher Diastolic-90 or higher **Hypotension** Systolic -90 mmHg or less

THE HEART: STRUCTURE, FUNCTION, AND CARDIAC EMERGENCIES

1. Structure of the Heart

The heart is a **muscular pump** that circulates blood throughout the body. It has **four chambers**:

Upper chambers (Atria)

Right atrium- The **right atrium** is one of the **four chambers of the heart**, located in the **upper right side**. Its key role is to **receive deoxygenated blood** from the body and pass it to the **right ventricle**, which then pumps it to the lungs for oxygenation.

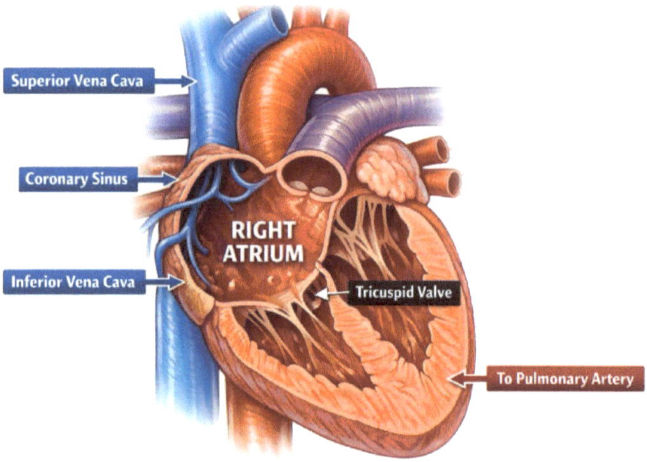

Left atrium-The **left atrium** is one of the four chambers of the heart. Its primary role is to **receive oxygen-rich blood from the lungs** via the pulmonary veins, then pump it into the left ventricle, which sends it to the rest of the body. Key points about the left atrium:

- **Location:** Upper left side of the heart.

- **Function:** Acts as a holding chamber for blood returning from the lungs.
- **Connection:** Blood flows from the left atrium through the **mitral valve** into the left ventricle.

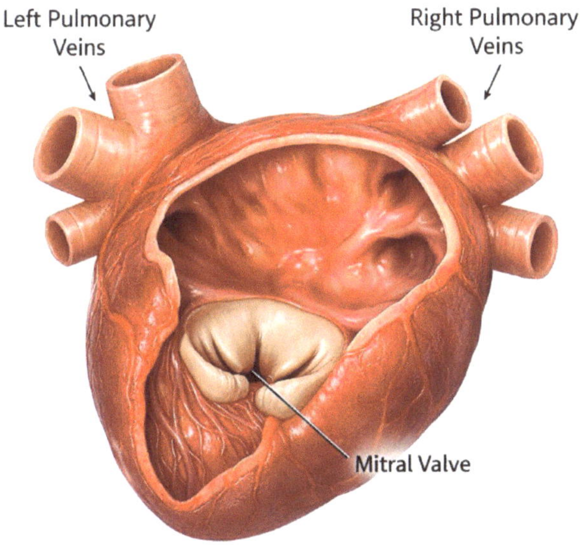

Left Atrium

Lower chambers (ventricles)

Right ventricle-The **right ventricle** is one of the four chambers of the heart.

In simple terms:

- It is the **lower right chamber** of the heart.
- Its job is to **pump deoxygenated (low oxygen) blood to the lungs**.

How it works:

1. Deoxygenated blood enters the **right atrium** from the body.
2. Blood flows from the right atrium into the **right ventricle**.
3. When the right ventricle contracts, it pumps blood through the **pulmonary valve** into the **pulmonary artery**.
4. The blood then travels to the **lungs**, where it picks up oxygen.

Key features:

- Has a **thinner muscular wall** than the left ventricle because it pumps blood at **lower pressure** (only to the lungs, not the whole body).
- Plays a vital role in **oxygenation of blood** and overall circulation.

Why it is important:
If the right ventricle fails, blood can back up in the body, causing symptoms such as **leg swelling, abdominal swelling, and breathlessness**.

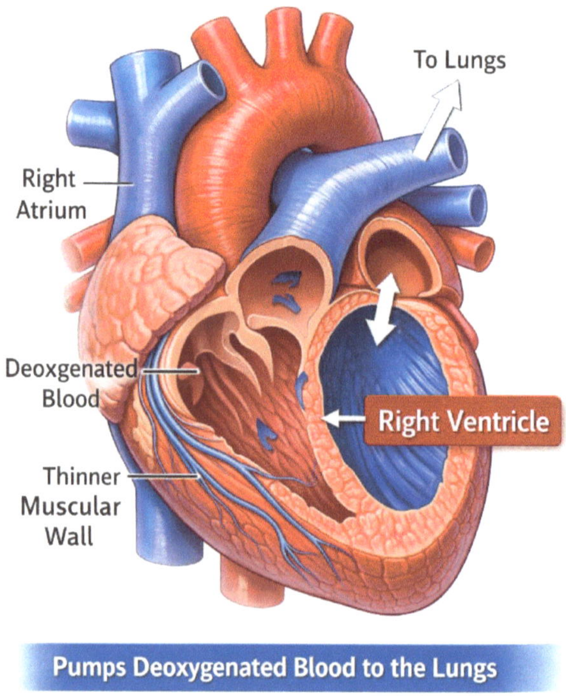

Left ventricle-The **left ventricle** is one of the four chambers of the heart. Its key role is to **pump oxygen-rich blood around the body**.

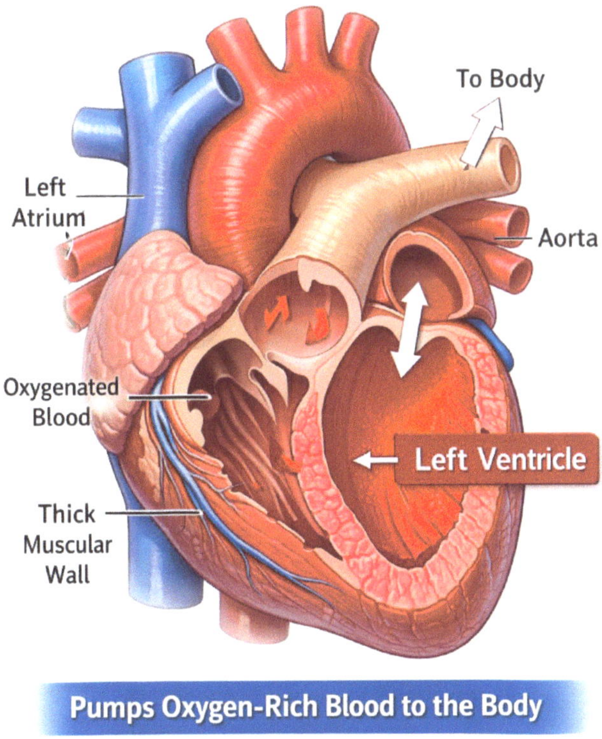

Key points:

- It receives oxygenated blood from the **left atrium**
- It pumps this blood into the **aorta**, the body's largest artery
- From the aorta, blood is delivered to all organs and tissues
- It has **thick muscular walls** because it must generate high pressure to circulate blood throughout the body

Why it is it important:

The left ventricle is the heart's main pumping chamber. If it does not work correctly, organs may not receive enough oxygen, leading to conditions such as **heart failure** or **shock**.

2. Function of the Right and Left Sides of the Heart

Right Side of the Heart

- Receives **deoxygenated blood** from the body.
- Pumps blood to the **lungs** for oxygenation via the pulmonary circulation.

Left Side of the Heart

- Receives **oxygenated blood** from the lungs
- Pumps blood to the **rest of the body** via the systemic circulation

3. Blood Vessels

- **Arteries** – carry blood **away from the heart** (usually oxygenated)
- ***Coronary arteries*** supply the heart muscle itself
- **Veins** – return **deoxygenated blood** to the heart
- **Capillaries** – tiny vessels where **oxygen and nutrient exchange** occur.

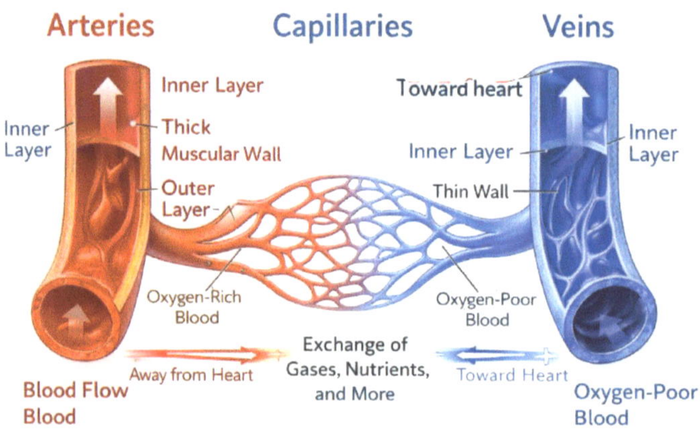

4. Heart Valves

Valves ensure **one-way blood flow** through the heart.

Right Side Valves

- **Tricuspid valve** – right atrium → right ventricle
- **Pulmonary valve** – right ventricle → lungs

Left Side Valves

- **Mitral (bicuspid) valve** – left atrium → left ventricle
- **Aortic valve** – left ventricle → aorta

5. Layers of the Heart

- **Pericardium** – protective outer sac
- **Myocardium** – muscular layer responsible for contraction
- **Endocardium** – smooth inner lining of chambers and valves

Septum

- Separates the left and right sides of the heart
- Prevents mixing of oxygenated and deoxygenated blood

6. How Oxygenated Blood Circulates

1. Right atrium receives deoxygenated blood
2. The right ventricle pumps blood to lungs
3. The left atrium receives oxygenated blood
4. The left ventricle pumps blood to the body

7. The Heart's Electrical (Conduction) System

The heart beats due to an internal electrical system:

- **Sinoatrial (SA) node** – natural pacemaker (60–100 bpm)
- **Atrioventricular (AV) node** – delays impulse to allow ventricular filling
- **Bundle of His** – transmits impulse to ventricles
- **Purkinje fibres** – coordinate ventricular contraction

Autonomic Control

- **Sympathetic system** – increases heart rate
- **Parasympathetic system** – slows heart rate

Cardiac Conduction System — Explained Simply and Clearly

The **cardiac conduction system** is the heart's **electrical wiring**. It controls **when and how the heart beats**, ensuring the chambers contract in the correct order to pump blood effectively.

1. Sinoatrial (SA) Node – *The natural pacemaker*

- Located in the **right atrium**
- Generates electrical impulses automatically
- Sets the normal heart rate (**60–100 bpm** in adults)
- Each impulse starts one heartbeat

This is why Normal Sinus Rhythm is called *sinus* rhythm.

2. Atrial Pathways

- Electrical impulse spreads across both atria
- Causes the **atria to contract**
- Pushes blood into the ventricles

This produces the **P wave** on the ECG.

3. Atrioventricular (AV) Node – *The delay point*

- Located between the atria and ventricles
- **Briefly delays** the electrical signal
- Allows ventricles time to fill with blood

The delay is vital for efficient cardiac output.

4. Bundle of His

- Conducts the impulse from the AV node into the ventricles
- Only a normal electrical connection between atria and ventricles

5. Right and Left Bundle Branches

- Run down the interventricular septum
- Carry impulses to each ventricle
- Left branch splits into anterior and posterior fascicles

6. Purkinje Fibres

- Spread rapidly through ventricular muscle
- Cause **strong, coordinated ventricular contraction**

This produces the **QRS complex** on the ECG.

ECG Summary

ECG Component	Electrical Event
P wave	Atrial depolarisation
PR interval	AV node delay
QRS complex	Ventricular depolarisation
T wave	Ventricular repolarisation

Clinical importance (Resuscitation context)

- Disruption can cause **bradycardia, tachycardia, heart block, VF, or VT**
- Cardiac arrest rhythms occur when this system **fails or becomes chaotic**
- Defibrillation aims to **reset abnormal conduction**

8. Cardiac Rhythms

Normal Sinus Rhythm (NSR) is the **normal, healthy heart rhythm**.

What it means:

- The heartbeat starts from the **sinoatrial (SA) node**, the heart's natural pacemaker.

- Electrical impulses travel through the heart in an **organised and predictable way**.

Key features:

- **Regular rhythm**
- **Heart rate: 60–100 beats per minute (bpm)** in adults
- Each heartbeat has:
    - A **P wave** (atrial contraction)
    - Followed by a **QRS complex** (ventricular contraction)
    - Then a **T wave** (ventricular relaxation)

Why it is not shockable:

- Defibrillation is used for **chaotic or disorganised rhythms** (e.g. ventricular fibrillation).
- Normal Sinus Rhythm is **organised**, so a shock would **not help and could be harmful**.

Clinical significance (basic life support context):

- If a patient has NSR, the heart is **electrically and mechanically functioning**.
- Cardiac arrest rhythms are **not NSR**.

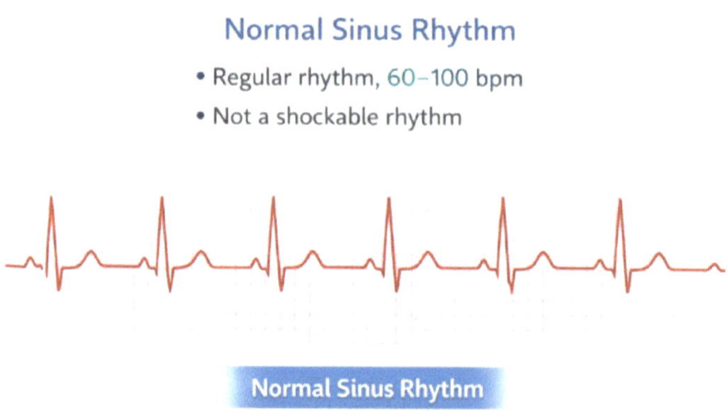

Ventricular Fibrillation (VF)

Ventricular fibrillation (VF) is a **life-threatening cardiac arrest rhythm**.

What it is

Ventricular fibrillation occurs when the **ventricles quiver chaotically instead of contracting normally**. The heart's electrical activity becomes completely disorganised, so **no effective cardiac output** is produced.

What happens in the heart

- Electrical impulses fire **randomly and rapidly**
- Ventricles **do not pump blood**
- **Circulation stops immediately**
- The person becomes **unconscious within seconds** and will die without rapid treatment

ECG characteristics

- **Chaotic, irregular waveform**
- **No identifiable P waves, QRS complexes, or T waves**
- May appear **coarse** (large waves) or **fine** (small waves)

Why it is shockable

- VF is caused by **disorganised electrical activity**
- **Defibrillation** delivers a controlled shock to:
    - Stop the chaotic activity
    - Allow the heart's natural pacemaker to restart a normal rhythm

Clinical importance (BLS / ALS context)

- VF is a **shockable cardiac arrest rhythm**
- Management includes:
    - **Immediate CPR**
    - **Early defibrillation**

- Advanced life support and reversible cause management (4 Hs & 4 Ts)

.

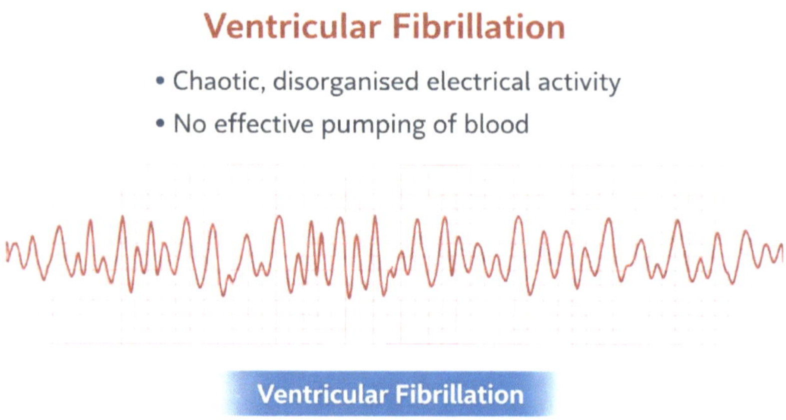

- Chaotic electrical activity
- **Shockable** rhythm

Pulseless Ventricular Tachycardia (VT)

Pulseless ventricular tachycardia (pVT) is a **life-threatening cardiac arrest rhythm** where the heart has electrical activity but **no effective cardiac output**.

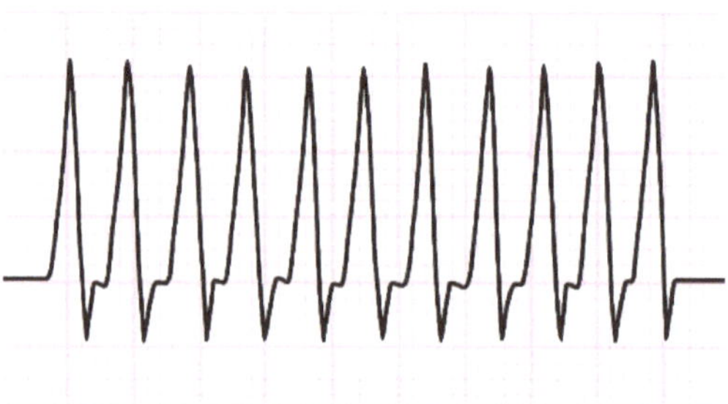

Pulseless Ventricular Tachycardia

What it is

This is a **fast, abnormal rhythm** originating from the **ventricles.**

The ventricles contract **so rapidly and inefficiently** that they **cannot fill or pump blood**. There is no **palpable pulse**, despite organised electrical activity.

→ The patient is in **cardiac arrest**.

ECG features

- **Regular, wide-complex tachycardia**
- Rate usually **>150–250 bpm**
- **No visible P waves**
- QRS complexes are **wide and uniform** (monomorphic) or variable (polymorphic)

Why there is no pulse

- Extreme rate → **no ventricular filling time**
- Poor coordination → **ineffective contraction**
- Cardiac output falls to **zero**

Why it is shockable

- pVT is caused by **organised but dangerous electrical activity**
- **Defibrillation** can interrupt the rhythm
- Allows the heart's natural pacemaker to re-establish control

pVT is a **shockable rhythm** (like VF)

Clinical presentation

- Unconscious
- Not breathing normally (or apnoeic)
- **No central pulse**
- Collapse may be sudden

Management (ALS overview)

- **Immediate CPR**
- **Defibrillation ASAP**
- Adrenaline and amiodarone per ALS algorithm
- Identify and treat **reversible causes (4 Hs & 4 Ts)**

Difference from VT with a pulse

Feature	VT with pulse	Pulseless VT
Pulse	Present	**Absent**
Blood pressure	Low/unstable	**None**
Consciousness	May be reduced	**Unconscious**
Management	Cardioversion/antiarrhythmics	**CPR + defibrillation**

Asystolic rhythm (Asystole)

Asystole is a **cardiac arrest rhythm** in which there is **no electrical activity in the heart**. It is commonly referred to as **"flatline."** Because there is no electrical impulse, there is **no cardiac contraction and no cardiac output**, making it a **medical emergency with an abysmal prognosis**.

Key characteristics

- **ECG appearance:** Near-flat line with no P waves, QRS complexes, or T waves
- **Heart activity:** None (no depolarisation)
- **Pulse:** Absent
- **Blood pressure:** Absent
- **Shockable rhythm:** No (defibrillation is not effective)

Common causes (Hs and Ts)

- **Hypoxia**

- **Severe acidosis**
- **Hypovolemia**
- **Electrolyte imbalance (especially potassium)**
- **Massive myocardial infarction**
- **Drug overdose**
- **Prolonged cardiac arrest**

Management

- Immediate **high-quality CPR**
- **Epinephrine** administration
- **Identify and treat reversible causes**
- Confirm rhythm is true asystole (check leads, gain, loose electrodes)

ECG illustration of asystole

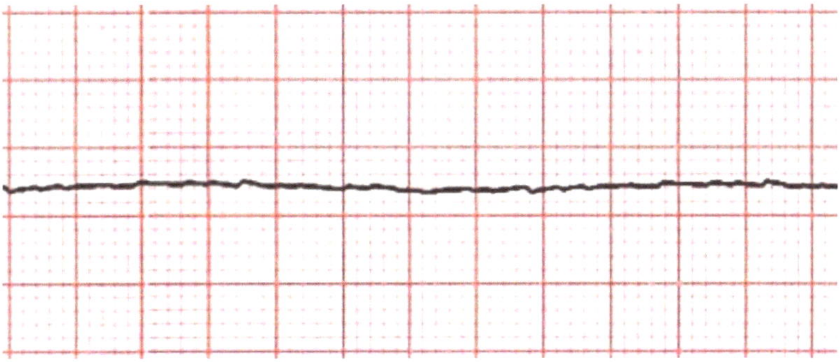

If you want, I can also **compare asystole with ventricular fibrillation or PEA**, or explain how to **distinguish true asystole from fine VF** on ECG.

9. Do Not Attempt Cardiopulmonary Resuscitation (DNACPR)

- Consent is assumed if a patient is unresponsive
- DNACPR applies **only to CPR**, not other treatments
- Treatment must follow legal and national guidance

Based on *Decisions Relating to Cardiopulmonary Resuscitation* (BMA, RCUK, RCN)

10. Acute Coronary Syndromes (ACS)

ACS describes conditions caused by **reduced blood flow to the heart muscle**:

- Stable angina
- Unstable angina
- Non-ST elevation myocardial infarction (NSTEMI)
- ST elevation myocardial infarction (STEMI)

Angina

Stable Angina

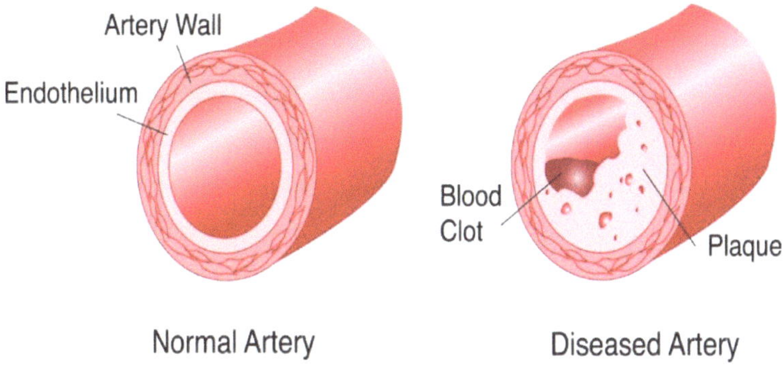

Stable angina is a type of **chest pain or discomfort** caused by **reduced blood flow to the heart muscle** (myocardial ischaemia), usually due to **coronary artery disease**.

What happens

- The coronary arteries are **narrowed by atherosclerosis**
- At rest, blood flow may be adequate
- During **exertion, stress, or cold**, the heart needs more oxygen
- The narrowed arteries **cannot meet this increased demand**
- This causes **temporary ischaemia → chest pain**

Key features (classic pattern)

- **Predictable**: occurs with the same level of exertion
- **Relieved by rest** or **glyceryl trinitrate (GTN)**
- Lasts **minutes (usually <10–15 minutes)**
- Does **not cause permanent heart damage**

Typical symptoms

- Central chest discomfort described as tightness, pressure, or heaviness

- Pain that may radiate to the left arm, neck, jaw, or back
- Common associated symptoms include:
    - Breathlessness
    - Sweating
    - Nausea
    - Fatigue

Common triggers

- Physical exertion
- Emotional stress
- Wintry weather
- Heavy meals

How it differs from unstable angina / MI

Feature	Stable Angina	Unstable Angina / MI
Pattern	Predictable	Unpredictable
Occurs at rest	No	Yes (often)
Relief	Rest / GTN	Often poor
Duration	Short	Prolonged
Myocardial damage	No	Possible / likely

Diagnosis (UK context)

- Clinical history is key
- ECG may be normal at rest
- Functional testing or CT coronary angiography per **NICE guidance**
- Troponin is **normal**

Management (overview)

Lifestyle:

- Smoking cessation
- Exercise
- Diet and weight management

Medication:

- **GTN** for symptom relief
- **Beta-blockers** or **calcium channel blockers**
- **Antiplatelets** (e.g. aspirin)
- **Statins**

Revascularisation if symptoms persist:

- PCI (stent)
- CABG

Stable angina = predictable exertional chest pain relieved by rest or GTN.

UNSTABLE ANGINA

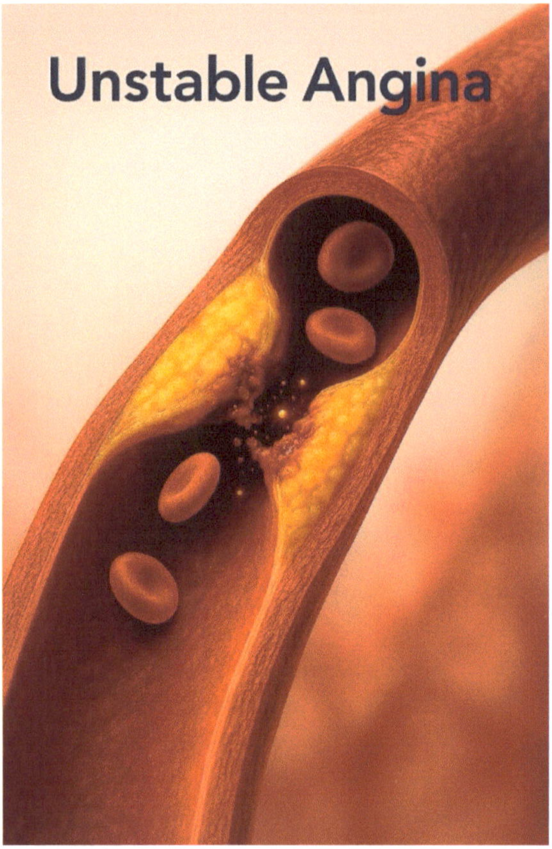

- Pain occurs at rest or worsening pattern
- Not reliably relieved by GTN
- Medical emergency

Common Symptoms

- Central chest pain radiating to the arm, jaw, neck, or back
- Breathlessness
- Nausea, dizziness, anxiety

Stable angina is predictable and occurs with exertion, while unstable angina is unpredictable, occurs even at rest, lasts longer, and is a medical emergency.

Key Differences Between Stable and Unstable Angina

Feature	Stable Angina	Unstable Angina
Pattern	Predictable, follows a consistent pattern	Unpredictable, no clear pattern
Triggers	Physical exertion, emotional stress, wintry weather, heavy meals	Can occur at rest, during sleep, or with minimal effort
Duration	Usually short (1–5 minutes, rarely >15 minutes)	Longer-lasting (>15–20 minutes, sometimes 30+ minutes)
Relief	Improves with rest or nitro-glycerine	May not improve with rest or medication
Severity	Less severe, manageable with lifestyle changes and medication	More severe, sudden worsening of symptoms
Urgency	Not usually an emergency, but requires medical follow-up	Always an emergency — immediate medical attention needed
Classification	Not part of acute coronary syndrome (ACS)	Classified as ACS (warning sign of a heart attack)
Cause	Narrowing of the coronary arteries due to plaque buildup	Plaque rupture and clot formation cause sudden reduced blood flow

Sources: Very well Health, Medicover Hospitals, Coppell ER

Why This Matters

- **Stable angina** is a chronic condition that can often be managed with medication, lifestyle changes, and monitoring.
- **Unstable angina** is a red flag for an impending heart attack. It reflects a sudden change in coronary artery disease and requires **emergency care**.

If chest pain is **new, worsening, occurs at rest, lasts longer than usual, or does not improve with nitroglycerine**, it should be treated as **unstable angina** and warrants **immediate emergency evaluation**.

Myocardial Infarction (Heart Attack)

A **heart attack**, medically called a **myocardial infarction (MI)**, happens when **blood flow to part of the heart muscle is suddenly blocked**, causing that portion of the heart muscle to be **damaged or die** due to lack of oxygen.

Main cause

The most common cause is **coronary artery disease**:

1. **Fatty plaques (atherosclerosis)** build up in the coronary arteries
2. A plaque **ruptures**
3. A **blood clot (thrombus)** forms on the rupture
4. The clot **blocks blood flow** to the heart muscle
5. Heart muscle downstream becomes **ischemic and necrotic**

What happens to the heart

- Oxygen deprivation begins within minutes
- Irreversible muscle damage can occur after **20–40 minutes**
- The affected heart muscle loses its ability to contract normally

Common symptoms

- Chest pain or pressure (often radiating to arm, jaw, or back)
- Shortness of breath
- Sweating, nausea, dizziness
- Fatigue (especially in women and older adults)

Illustration: cause of a heart attack

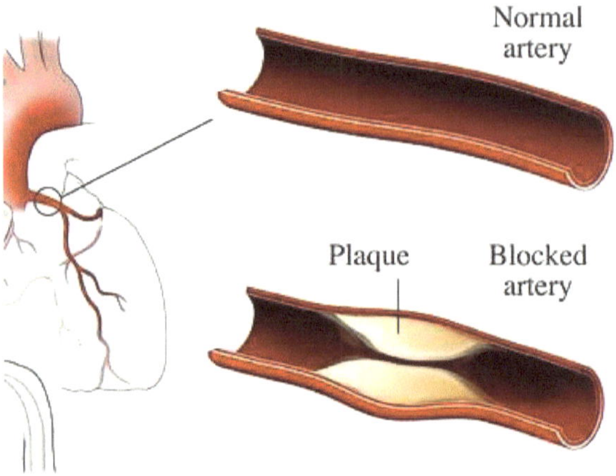

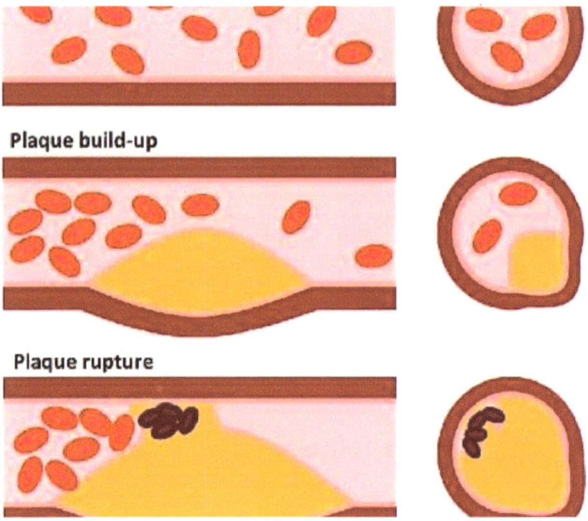

Key point to remember

A heart attack is **not** caused by the heart "stopping," but by **blocked blood supply** to the heart muscle.

STEMI vs NSTEMI (Types of Heart Attacks)

Both **STEMI** and **NSTEMI** are forms of **acute myocardial infarction (AMI)**, meaning heart muscle damage caused by reduced blood flow. The key difference lies in the **degree of coronary artery blockage and ECG findings**.

STEMI

ST-Elevation Myocardial Infarction

What happens

- **Complete (or near-complete) blockage** of a coronary artery
- Causes **full-thickness (transmural) myocardial infarction**

ECG findings

- **ST-segment elevation** in **≥2 contiguous leads**
- May later develop **pathologic Q waves**

Cardiac enzymes

- **Troponin: elevated**

Treatment urgency

🚨 **Immediate reperfusion required**

- Primary **PCI (angioplasty/stent)** preferred
- **Thrombolytics** if PCI unavailable

NSTEMI

Non-ST-Elevation Myocardial Infarction

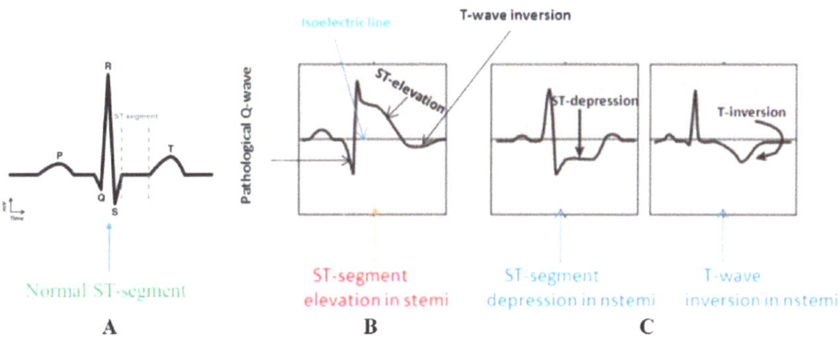

What happens

- **Partial or intermittent blockage** of a coronary artery
- Causes **partial-thickness (subendocardial) infarction**

ECG findings

- **No ST elevation**
- May show:
    - **ST depression**
    - **T-wave inversion**
    - Or **normal ECG**

Cardiac enzymes

- **Troponin: elevated**

Treatment urgency

Urgent but not immediate reperfusion

- Antiplatelets, anticoagulants
- Early invasive strategy (angiography within 24–72 hrs)

STEMI occurs when a coronary artery is completely blocked, leading to full-thickness heart muscle damage.

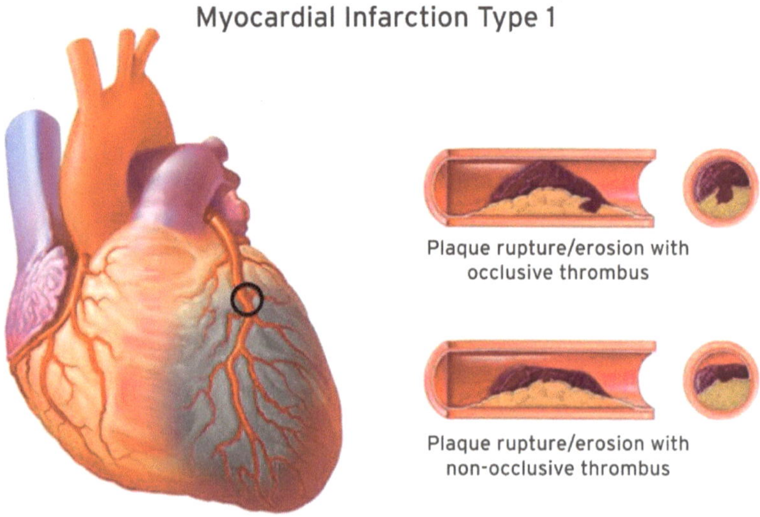

NSTEMI (Non–ST-Elevation Myocardial Infarction)

NSTEMI is a type of **heart attack** in which there is **heart muscle damage due to reduced blood flow**, but **without ST-segment elevation on the ECG**.

What happens in NSTEMI

- A **coronary artery is partially or intermittently blocked**
- Blood flow is **reduced, not completely stopped**
- Causes **partial-thickness (subendocardial) damage** to the heart muscle

ECG findings

- **No ST elevation**
- May show:
  - **ST-segment depression**
  - **T-wave inversion**
  - Or even a **normal ECG**

Blood tests

- **Cardiac troponins: elevated** (confirms myocardial injury)

How NSTEMI differs from STEMI

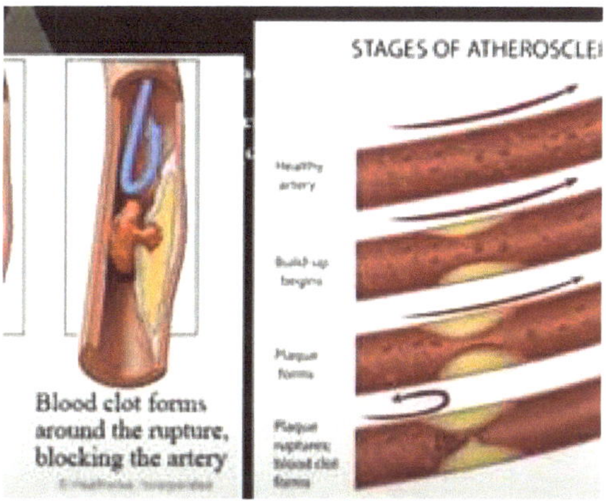

Feature	NSTEMI	STEMI
Artery blockage	Partial	Complete

Feature	NSTEMI	STEMI
ST elevation	No	Yes
Heart muscle damage	Partial thickness	Full thickness
Immediate PCI	Usually not immediate	Immediate

NSTEMI = heart attack with elevated troponin but no ST elevation, usually due to partial coronary artery blockage.

Difference Between NSTEMI and Unstable Angina

Both **NSTEMI** and **unstable angina (UA)** are forms of **acute coronary syndrome (ACS)** and often look similar clinically.
The **key difference** is **heart muscle damage**, as measured by **cardiac troponin levels**.

NSTEMI (Non–ST-Elevation Myocardial Infarction)

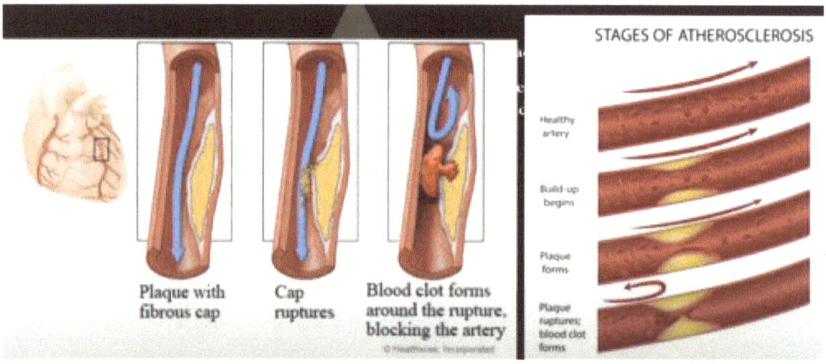

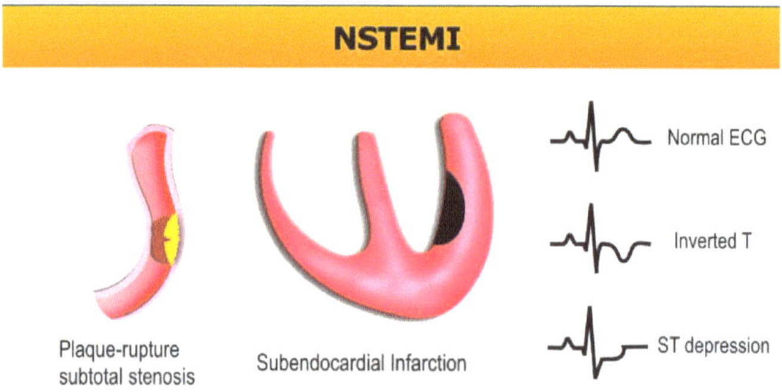

What happens

- **Partial or intermittent coronary artery blockage**
- Causes **irreversible myocardial cell death**

ECG

- No ST elevation
- May show **ST depression or T-wave inversion**

Troponin

- **Elevated**

Unstable Angina

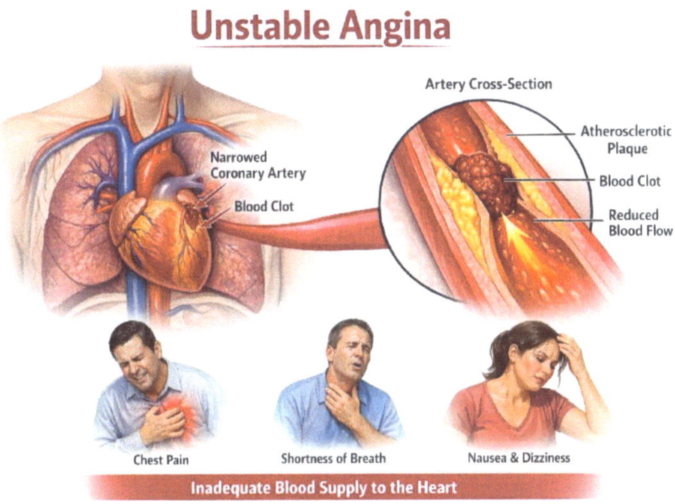

What happens

- **Transient or incomplete ischemia**
- **No myocardial cell death**

ECG

- Normal or **transient ST depression/T-wave inversion**

Troponin

- **Normal**

Side-by-side comparison

Feature	NSTEMI	Unstable Angina
Coronary blockage	Partial	Partial/transient
Myocardial damage	Yes (infarction)	No
Troponin	**Elevated**	**Normal**
ECG	ST ↓ / T inversion	Normal or transient changes
Prognosis	Worse than UA	Better than NSTEMI

High-yield clinical rule

Troponin elevated = NSTEMI
Troponin normal = Unstable angina

STEMI vs NSTEMI — Quick comparison

Feature	STEMI	NSTEMI
Coronary blockage	Complete	Partial
ST elevation on ECG	Yes	No
Troponin	Elevated	Elevated
Heart muscle damage	Full thickness	Partial thickness
Immediate PCI	Required	Not immediate

ST elevation = total occlusion = immediate Cath lab

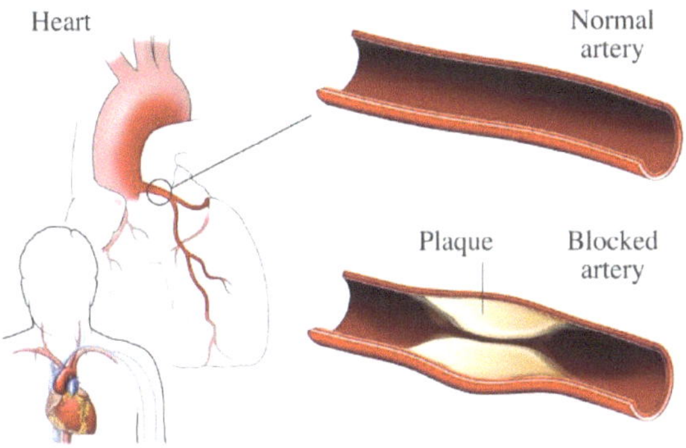

Occurs due to **coronary artery blockage**, leading to heart muscle death.

Symptoms

- Persistent crushing chest pain (>15 minutes)
- Breathlessness
- Nausea or vomiting
- Pale, clammy skin
- Sense of impending doom

Emergency Medications

Glyceryl Trinitrate (GTN)

Indication: Suspected angina or MI if systolic BP ≥90 mmHg

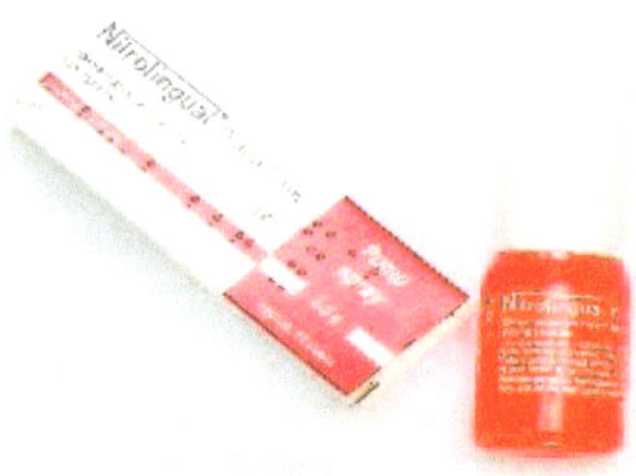

- Spray: 400 micrograms sublingually
- Repeat every 5 minutes if required

Contraindications:

- Hypotension
- Recent PDE-5 inhibitors (e.g. sildenafil within 24–48h)
- Head injury or intracranial haemorrhage

Side effects: Headache, dizziness, hypotension

Aspirin

Indication: Suspected ACS

- Adult dose: **300 mg orally (chewed or dissolved)**

Do NOT give if:

- Known aspirin allergy

- Active GI bleeding

Caution (benefit usually outweighs risk):

- Asthma, pregnancy, renal disease

SUDDEN CARDIAC ARREST (SCA)

Sudden cardiac arrest occurs when the heart **abruptly stops pumping blood effectively**, leading to **loss of cardiac output, loss of consciousness, and absence of a pulse**. Without immediate treatment, it is **rapidly fatal**.

Survival

- Overall survival to hospital discharge in out-of-hospital cardiac arrest is **8–10%**
- Survival depends on:
  - **Early recognition**
  - **Immediate high-quality CPR**
  - **Early defibrillation (if shockable rhythm)**
  - **Rapid advanced life support and post-resuscitation care**

Chain of Prevention in a Dental Setting

1. Identify Risk Early

- Take a thorough medical history at every visit
- Identify high-risk patients (e.g. cardiac disease, diabetes, asthma, allergies)
- Reduce triggers: anxiety, pain, dehydration, prolonged supine positioning

2. Prepare the Team

- All staff trained in **BLS, AED use, and medical emergencies**
- Annual updates and regular practice drills
- Clear roles agreed in advance (who calls 999, who starts CPR, who gets the AED)

3. Prepare the Environment

- Emergency drugs and equipment immediately accessible
- AED available on site
- Oxygen, suction, airway equipment checked regularly and documented

4. Recognise Deterioration Early

- Use **ABCDE approach** for unwell patients
- Recognise red flags: collapse, unresponsiveness, abnormal breathing
- Act early — do not wait for cardiac arrest

5. Respond Immediately

- Call **999 or 112** early
- Start **high-quality CPR** if cardiac arrest is suspected
- Use the **AED as soon as it is available**
- Follow dispatcher instructions until help arrives

6. Review & Learn

- Handover clearly to the ambulance crew
- Debrief the team after the event
- Update training, protocols, and equipment checks as needed

Good prevention = good preparation.
Early risk assessment, trained staff, ready equipment, and fast action save lives.

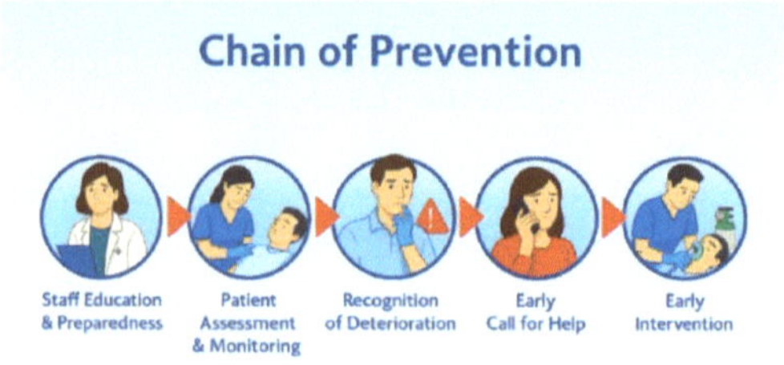

CAUSES OF CARDIAC ARREST

According to the **Resuscitation Council UK (ALS)**, causes should be systematically considered using the **Reversible Causes: the 4 Hs and 4 Ts**.

The 4 Hs

Hypoxia

- Most common cause
- From airway obstruction, respiratory failure, asthma, pneumonia, opioid overdose

Hypovolaemia

- Severe blood or fluid loss
- Trauma, GI bleeding, dehydration, sepsis

Hypo-/Hyperkalaemia (and other metabolic disturbances)

- Electrolyte imbalance (especially potassium)
- Diabetic ketoacidosis (DKA)
- Renal failure

Hypothermia

- Core temperature <35°C
- Reduced cardiac excitability and contractility

The 4 Ts

Tension pneumothorax

- Air trapped under pressure in pleural space
- Compresses heart and lungs → obstructive shock

Cardiac tamponade

- Fluid/blood in pericardial sac
- Prevents ventricular filling

Toxins

- Drug overdose (opioids, TCAs, beta-blockers, calcium channel blockers)
- Poisoning

Thrombosis

- **Coronary thrombosis** → acute myocardial infarction
- **Pulmonary thrombosis** → massive pulmonary embolism

Common clinical conditions leading to cardiac arrest

(Integrated into Hs and Ts per guidelines)

- **Myocardial infarction** → Coronary thrombosis
- **Pulmonary embolism** → Pulmonary thrombosis
- **Diabetic ketoacidosis** → Metabolic disturbance (H)
- **Sepsis** → Hypovolaemia, hypoxia, metabolic acidosis
- **Severe asthma** → Hypoxia
- **Hypothermia** → Hypothermia (H)

Key NICE & RCUK principles

- Cardiac arrest management prioritises:
    - **Immediate CPR**
    - **Early defibrillation for shockable rhythms (VF/pVT)**
    - **Rapid identification and treatment of reversible causes**
- **Asystole and PEA are non-shockable rhythms**
- Treating the **underlying cause** is essential for survival

Summary

Sudden cardiac arrest = sudden loss of cardiac output
Think 4 Hs and 4 Ts
Early CPR and defibrillation save lives

DENTAL RESUSCITATION EQUIPMENT REQUIREMENTS

Defibrillation Equipment

- **Automated External Defibrillator (AED)**
    - Must be **immediately accessible** in all clinical areas where patients are seen, including:
        - Dentists
        - Dental hygienists or therapists
        - Dental technicians (if treating patients)
        - Any combination of dental team members
- The AED must be:
    - Clearly visible
    - **Indicated with standard AED signage**
    - Checked regularly and maintained according to manufacturer instructions

Defibrillator Accessories

- **Adhesive defibrillator pads**
    - Adult pads (mandatory)
    - **Spare set of pads strongly recommended**
- **Scissors**
- **Razor** (for chest hair removal if required)

Emergency Drug Kit

- An **appropriate emergency drug kit** must be available **on-site** in dental practices where clinicians are permitted to administer medicines.
- Drugs should align with current **RCUK dental emergency recommendations** (e.g. for anaphylaxis, hypoglycaemia, asthma, cardiac arrest).

- Drugs must be:
    - In-date
    - Clearly labelled
    - Easily accessible
- Staff must be trained in:
    - Indications
    - Doses
    - Routes of administration

Oxygen and Airway Management Equipment

Oxygen Supply

- Each practice should have:
    - A **CD-size integral valve oxygen cylinder**
    - Capacity: **approximately 460 litres**
    - Capable of delivering:
        - **15 litres/minute**
        - For **approximately 30 minutes**
- Oxygen cylinders must be:
    - Securely stored
    - Regularly checked
    - Immediately available

Oxygen Delivery Equipment

- Oxygen tubing
- Oxygen masks with a reservoir
- Clear face masks compatible with self-inflating bags

Ventilation Equipment

- **Self-inflating bag with reservoir (adult)**

- **Self-inflating bag with reservoir (child)**
- **Clear face masks** for self-inflating bags:
    - Sizes **0, 1, 2, 3, and 4**

Airway Adjuncts

Oropharyngeal airways

- A full set of **7 sizes**:
    - 000, 00, 0, 1, 2, 3, 4

- **Pocket face masks**
    - A set of **5 clear pocket masks**, sizes **1–5**
    - Must include an **oxygen port**
    - Available **immediately within the first minutes** of a cardiac arrest

Suction Equipment

- **Portable suction device**
    - Must be:
        - Immediately available
        - Functional
        - Suitable for clearing airway secretions during resuscitation

Personal Protective Equipment (PPE)

The following must be available **immediately** in the event of cardiac arrest:

- Gloves
- Aprons
- Eye protection

Dental Technicians (CDTs) – Regulatory Clarification

Under the **Human Medicines Regulations 2012**:

- **Clinical Dental Technicians (CDTs)**:

    - Are **not permitted** to purchase or hold **prescription-only medicines**
    - Are **not required** to have an emergency drug kit
    - Are **not expected** to be trained in the use of emergency drugs
- The **Care Quality Commission (CQC)** does **not expect**:
    - Independently working CDTs
    - Or CDT-only premises
      to hold emergency drugs on-site

Key Compliance Points (CQC & RCUK)

- Equipment must be:
    - Immediately accessible
    - Regularly checked and documented
- Staff must:
    - Receive **annual training** in basic life support
    - Be familiar with the location and use of all resuscitation equipment
- Practices should conduct:
    - Regular **emergency drills**
    - Routine audits of emergency equipment

CQC Inspection Checklist – Dental Resuscitation Equipment & Preparedness

Practice Name: ___________________________
Practice Address: _________________________
Inspection / Audit Date: __________________
Responsible Lead: ________________________

1. Defibrillation Equipment

☐ **AED available on-site**

☐ AED is **immediately accessible** in all clinical areas

☐ AED location is **clearly visible**

☐ **Standard AED signage** in place

AED Accessories

☐ Adult adhesive defibrillator pads present

☐ **Spare set of pads available**

☐ Pads **in date**

☐ Scissors available

☐ Razor available (for chest hair removal)

Maintenance

☐ AED checked regularly

☐ Battery status checked and functional

☐ Maintenance log completed and up to date

2. Emergency Drug Kit

(Not applicable to CDT-only practices)

☐ Emergency drug kit present on-site

☐ Drugs align with **RCUK dental emergency recommendations**

☐ Drugs clearly labelled

☐ All drugs **in date**

☐ Drugs stored securely and accessible

☐ Staff trained in indications and administration

3. Oxygen Supply

☐ CD-size integral valve oxygen cylinder available

☐ Cylinder capacity approx. **460 litres**

☐ Capable of delivering **15 L/min**

☐ Cylinder sufficiently full

☐ Oxygen cylinder securely stored

☐ Regular checks documented

4. Oxygen Delivery Equipment

☐ Oxygen tubing available

☐ Oxygen masks with reservoir available

☐ Equipment clean and functional

5. Ventilation Equipment

☐ Adult self-inflating bag with reservoir

☐ Child self-inflating bag with reservoir

☐ Bags and reservoirs intact and functional

Face Masks

☐ Clear face masks compatible with bag-valve device

☐ Sizes available: 0 ☐ 1 ☐ 2 ☐ 3 ☐ 4 ☐

6. Airway Adjuncts

☐ Oropharyngeal airway set available

☐ Full set of sizes present:

- ☐ 000
- ☐ 00
- ☐ 0
- ☐ 1
- ☐ 2
- ☐ 3
- ☐ 4

☐ Airway adjuncts clean and in good condition

7. Pocket Face Masks

☐ Pocket face masks immediately available

☐ Total of **5 masks** present

☐ Sizes 1–5 available

☐ Masks include **oxygen port**

☐ Masks clean and functional

8. Suction Equipment

☐ Portable suction device available

☐ Suction immediately accessible

☐ Device tested and functional

☐ Suction catheters available

☐ Maintenance checks documented

9. Personal Protective Equipment (PPE)

☐ Gloves available

☐ Aprons available

☐ Eye protection available

☐ PPE immediately accessible during emergencies

10. Staff Training & Awareness

☐ All clinical staff trained in **Basic Life Support (BLS)**

☐ Training updated **annually**

☐ Staff trained in use of AED

☐ Staff aware of location of resuscitation equipment

☐ Emergency drills conducted

☐ Training records available

11. Dental Technicians (CDTs) – Regulatory Compliance

☐ CDT-only practice identified (if applicable)

☐ No prescription-only medicines held by CDTs

☐ Emergency drug kit **not required** for CDT-only practices

☐ Staff aware of scope of practice limitations

12. Documentation & Governance

☐ Emergency equipment checklist completed regularly

☐ Equipment checks documented

☐ Expiry dates monitored

☐ Policies align with **RCUK & NICE guidance**

☐ Evidence available for CQC inspection

Inspector / Auditor Comments

Action Plan (if required)

Issue Identified	Action Required	Responsible Person	Target Date

---

Audit Outcome

☐ Fully compliant

☐ Partially compliant (action required)

☐ Non-compliant (urgent action required)

Auditor Name & Signature: ____________________________
Date: ____________________

AIRWAY MANAGEMENT

USING THE I-GEL SUPRAGLOTTIC AIRWAY DEVICE

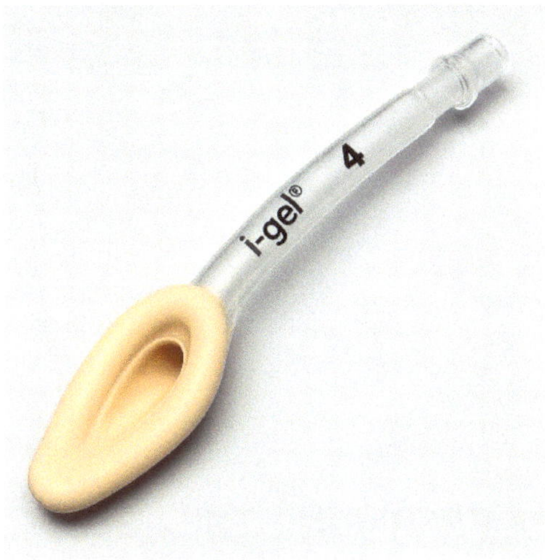

STEP 1-Choose the correct size and inspect the device

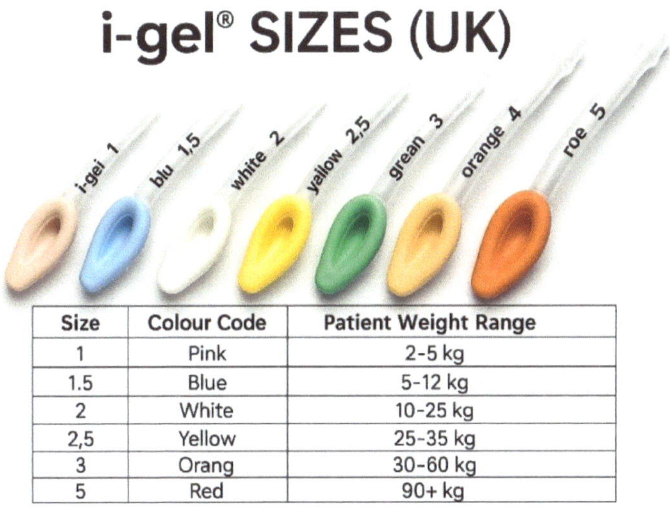

Size	Colour Code	Patient Weight Range
1	Pink	2-5 kg
1.5	Blue	5-12 kg
2	White	10-25 kg
2,5	Yellow	25-35 kg
3	Orang	30-60 kg
5	Red	90+ kg

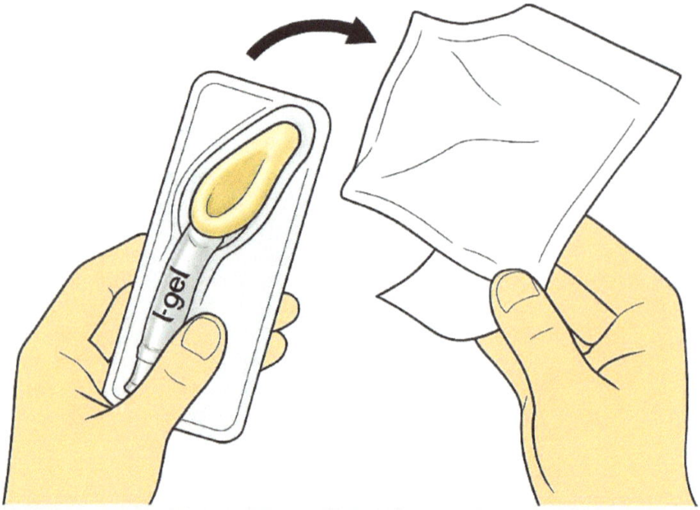

STEP 2 - PREPARING THE I-GEL FOR USE

Open the i-gel packaging and remove the protective cradle containing the device.

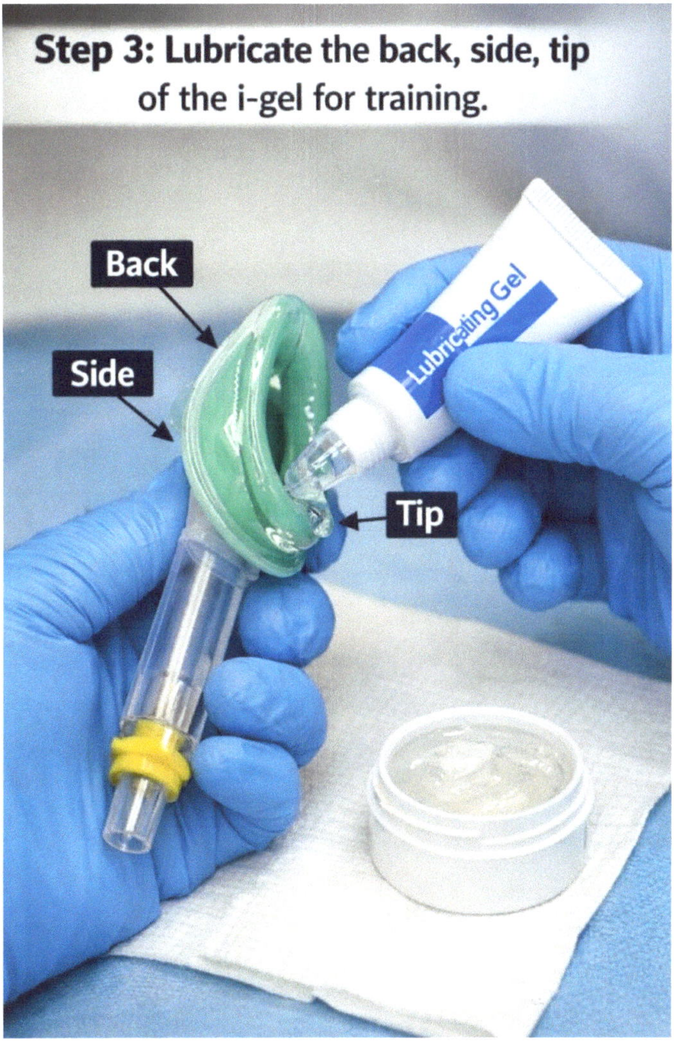
Step 3: Lubricate the back, side, tip
of the i-gel for training.
Back
Side
Tip
Lubricating Gel

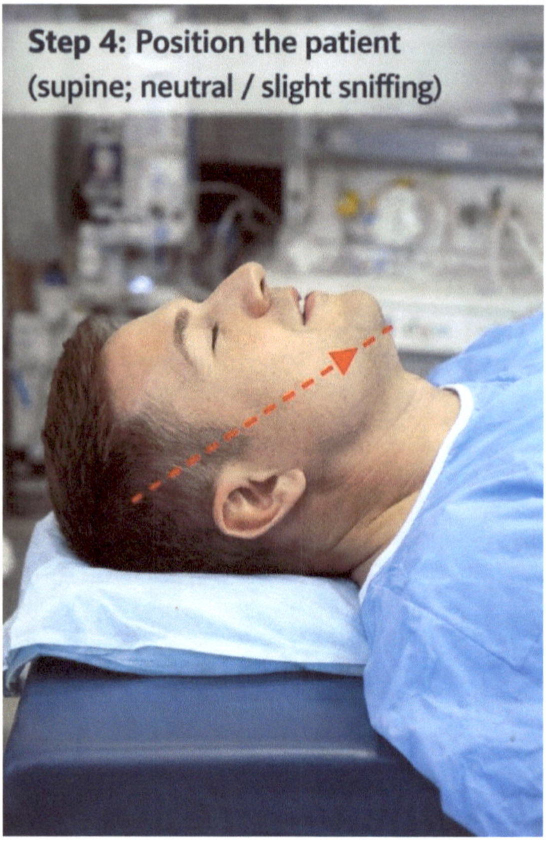
Step 4: Position the patient
(supine; neutral / slight sniffing)

STEP 5- OPEN THE MOUTH AND HOLD THE I-GEL BY THE BITE BLOCK;

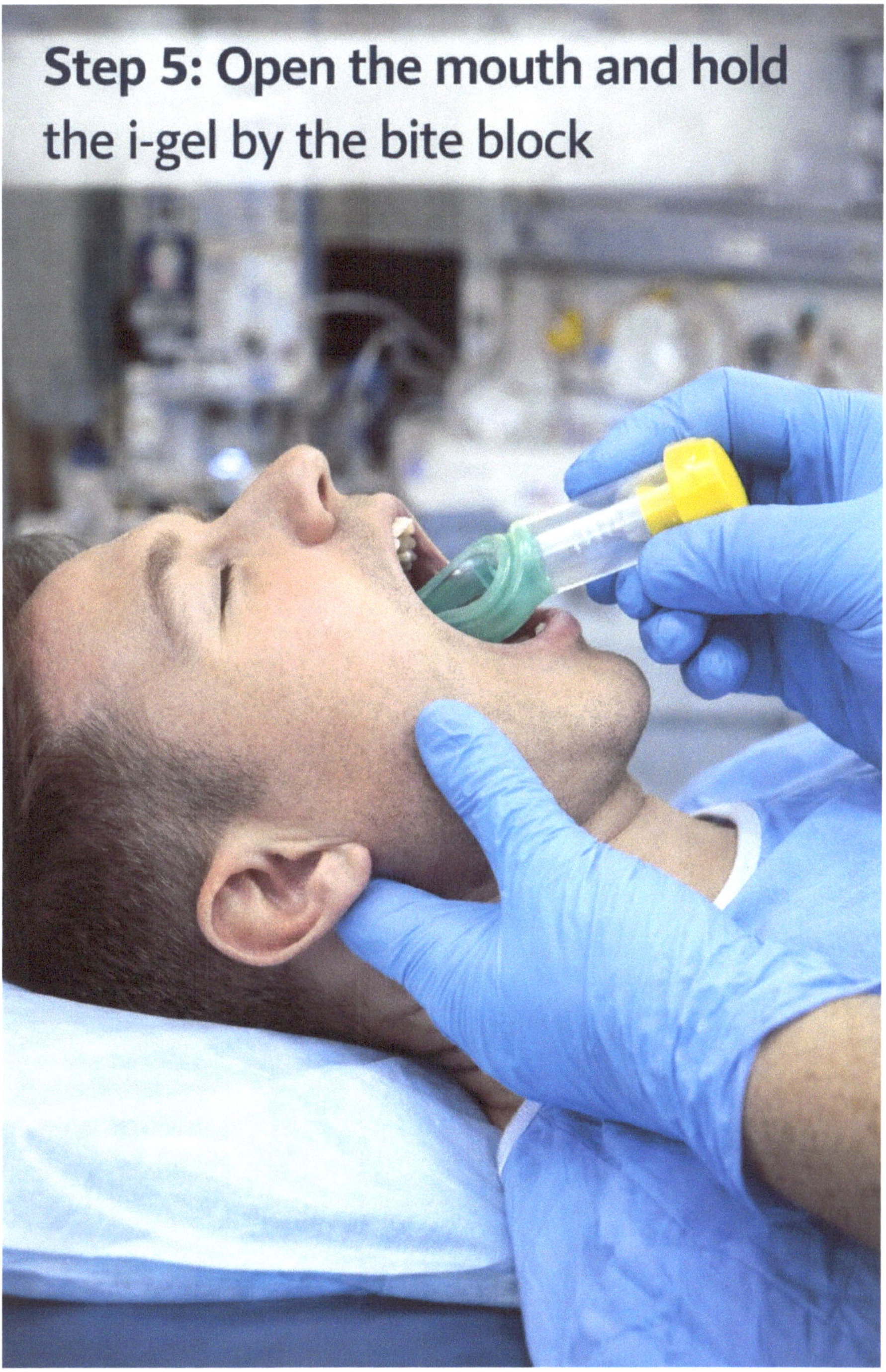

STEP 6-ADVANCE ALONG THE HARD PALATE IN A SMOOTH AND CONTINUOUS MOVEMENT UNTIL DEFINITE RESISTANCE IS FELT (THIS IS TYPICALLY THE CORRECT DEPTH

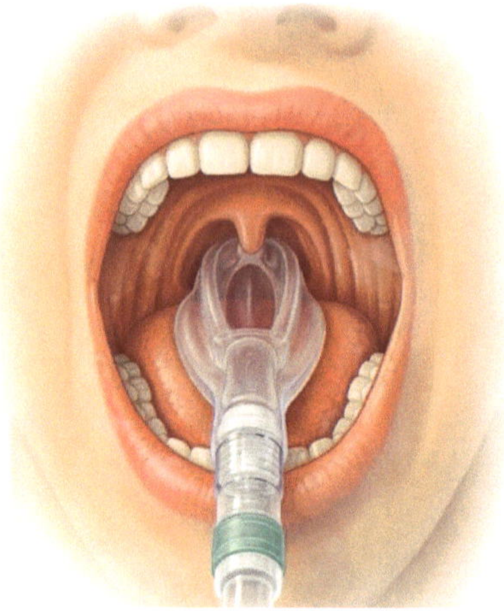

STEP 7: VENTILATE AND CONFIRM PLACEMENT: VISIBLE CHEST RISE,

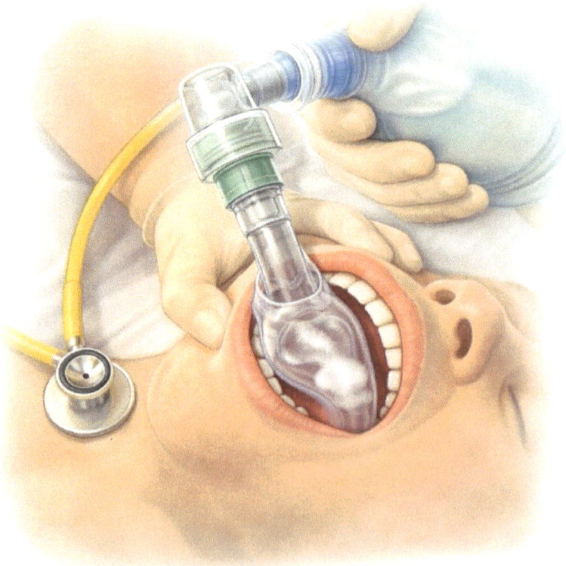

STEP 8: SECURE WITH TAPE STRAP AND CONTINUE MONITORING

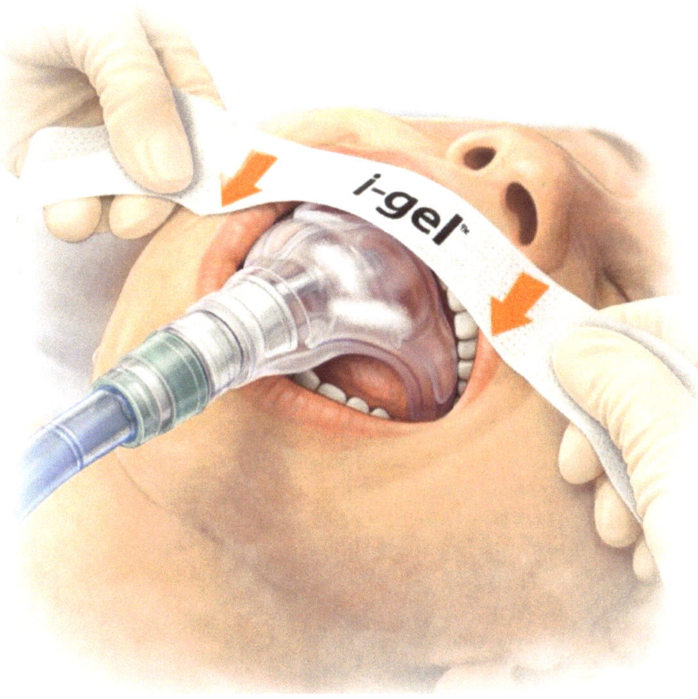

OROPHARYNGEAL AIRWAY

What is an OPA?

An **oropharyngeal airway (OPA)** is a rigid, curved plastic device inserted into the mouth to **keep the airway open** by preventing the tongue from falling back and blocking the throat.
It sits **over the tongue** in the **oropharynx** (back of the mouth).

Key Features

- Rigid, curved plastic device
- Inserted through the **mouth**
- Outer **flange** prevents it slipping inside
- Available in multiple sizes (infant, child, adult)
- Used to maintain airway patency in **unconscious patients**

When to Use an OPA

Use an OPA when:

- Patient is **unconscious**
- **No gag reflex** is present
- Tongue is causing airway obstruction
- Airway support is needed during **CPR**
- **Bag–valve–mask (BVM)** ventilation is required

When NOT to Use an OPA

Do **not** use an OPA if:

- Patient is **conscious or semi-conscious**
- Gag reflex is present (risk of vomiting or laryngospasm)
- Significant **oral trauma**, swelling, or obstruction exists

1. Indications & Safety

Check before insertion:

- Patient is unconscious
- No gag reflex (no coughing or retching)
- Airway obstruction risk from the tongue

Do NOT use if:

- Patient is conscious or semi-conscious
- Strong gag reflex present
- Major oral trauma or obstruction

Safety precautions:

- Wear gloves (eye protection if required)
- Ensure scene safety (D in **DRABCDE**)

2. Choosing the Correct Size (Very Important)

Sizing Methods

Measure:

- **Corner of the mouth → angle of the jaw**, **OR**
- **Incisors → angle of the mandible (or earlobe)**

Correct Size Check

- Flange rests at the **lips**
- Tip reaches the **angle of the jaw**

Why Sizing Matters

- **Too small:** pushes tongue backwards → worsens obstruction
- **Too large:** presses on epiglottis → gagging, trauma, vomiting
- **Correct size:** keeps airway open and allows effective ventilation

3. Prepare the Patient

- **Position head**
    - Head tilt–chin lift (if no trauma)
    - Jaw thrust if trauma suspected
- **Open the mouth**
    - Use scissor technique (thumb on lower incisors, finger on upper)

4. Insertion Technique

Adults

1. Hold OPA **upside down** (curve facing the roof of the mouth)
2. Insert along the **hard palate**
3. Rotate **180°** at the soft palate
4. Advance gently until the flange rests on the lips

Children & Infants

- **Do NOT rotate**
- Insert the OPA **right way up**
- Use a tongue depressor to move the tongue forward gently

5. Confirm Placement

- Flange sits comfortably against the lips
- OPA follows the natural curve of the tongue
- Improved airflow:
    - Better chest rise
    - Reduced snoring or gurgling sounds

If gagging or coughing occurs:

- Remove the OPA immediately
- Reassess airway and use basic airway manoeuvres

6. Ongoing Care

- Support airway with **BVM ventilation** if needed
- Reassess airway regularly as part of **DRABCDE**
- Monitor level of consciousness and breathing
- Document:
  - Size used
  - Time of insertion
  - Patient response

OPAs are **only for unconscious patients without a gag reflex**
Correct sizing and technique are critical
Continuous monitoring is essential

Why OPA sizing matters

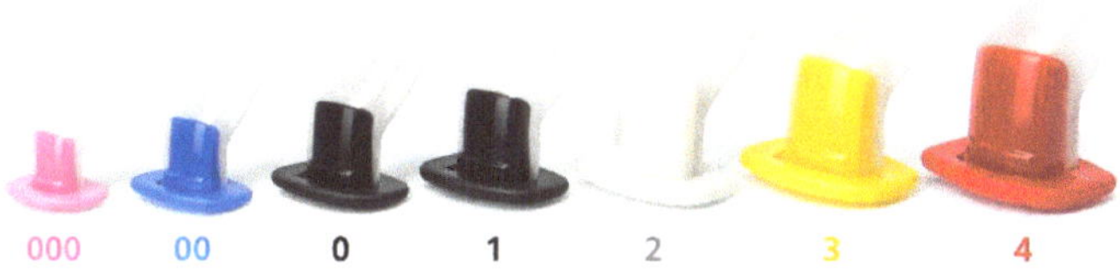

Choosing the right size of the OPA matters because the wrong size can obstruct the airway or cause injury:

Too small: Pushes the tongue backwards, worsening obstruction

Too large: presses on the epiglottis, gagging, trauma, vomiting

Correct size: keeps the airway open, allows ventilation, and allows effective airway management

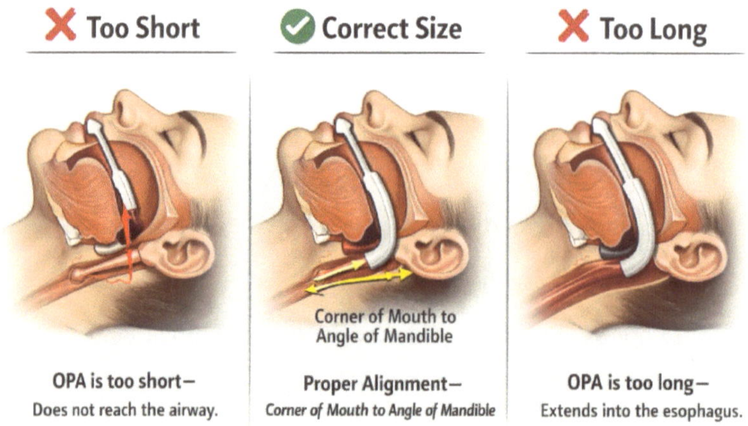

THE SIZING METHODS

Corner of the mouth to angle of the Jaw

Or from incisors to the earlobe

INSERTING THE OPA

Overview

- **Purpose:** Maintain airway patency in an unconscious patient with no gag reflex.
- **Applies to:** Any age group (adjust size selection per patient).

Step 1 – Prepare and position the patient

Text for learners:

- **Check safety:** Ensure scene safety and standard precautions.
- **Position:** Place the patient supine on a firm surface.

Head position: Open the airway with a head tilt–chin lift (unless suspected cervical spine injury).

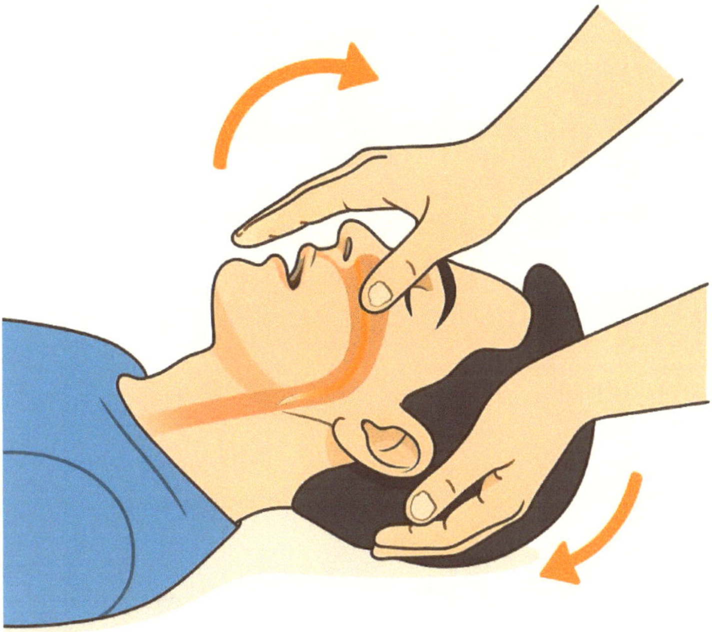

Step 2 – Select the correct OPA size

Text for learners:

- **Measure:** Align the OPA alongside the face.
    - From the **centre of the incisors** (or corner of the mouth) to the **angle of the mandible**.
- **Rule:** The flange should reach the incisors when the tip reaches the jaw angle.
- **Message:** Too small will not keep the airway open; too big may traumatise or obstruct.

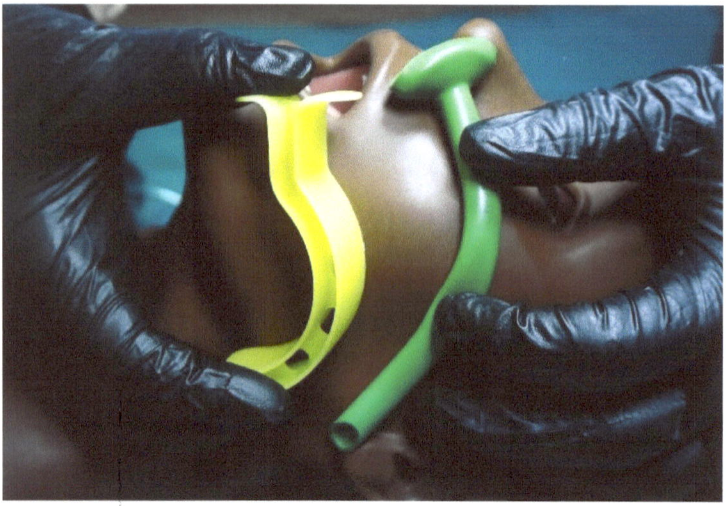

Step 3 – Inspect the mouth

Text for learners:

- **Check:** Open the mouth and quickly inspect for obvious obstructions.
- **Remove:** Use a finger sweep only if you can clearly see and safely remove visible solid material.
- **Avoid:** Blind finger sweeps, which can push material deeper.

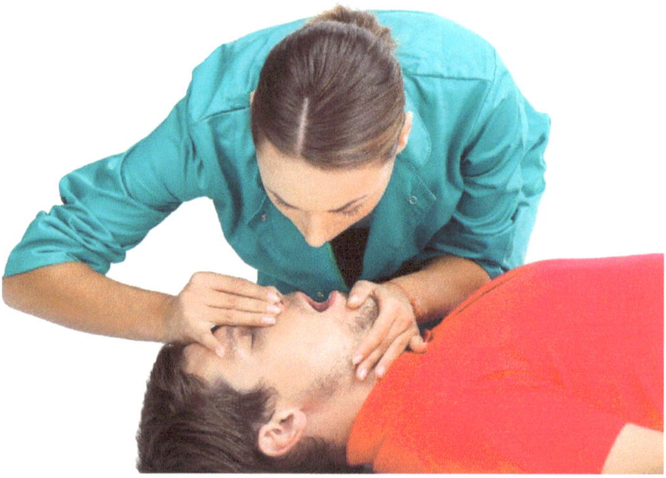

Step 4 – Insert the OPA (adult technique)

Text for learners:

- **Initial position:** Hold the OPA with the curve facing **upwards** (towards the roof of the mouth).
- **Entry:**
  - Insert the tip into the mouth along the hard palate.
  - Follow the contour of the palate to the soft palate.
- **Rotation:** Once the tip reaches the soft palate/oropharynx:
  - Rotate the OPA **180°** so the curve now follows the tongue.
- **Advance:** Gently advance until the flange rests on the lips/teeth.

OPA Rotation

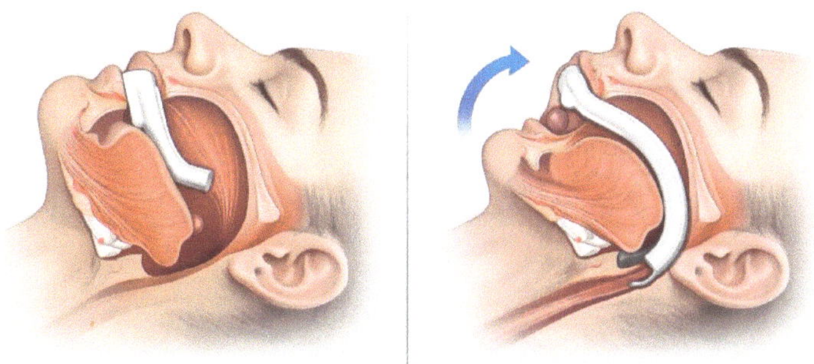

Frame 1: OPA tip at the soft palate

Frame 2: OPA rotated 180°

Step 5 – Alternative insertion (paediatric or when trauma risk)

- **Issue:** In children and some adults, rotation can cause soft tissue trauma or push the tongue back.
- **Alternative method:**
  - Insert the OPA **right way up from the start** (concavity facing the tongue).
  - Use a tongue depressor or your gloved fingers to gently hold the tongue forward.

- Slide the OPA in following the tongue's curve until the flange rests on the lips.

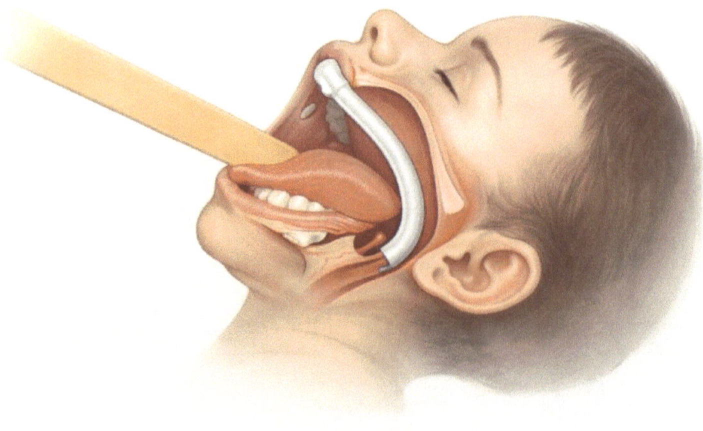

Step 6 – Confirm positioning

- **Flange:** Should rest comfortably against the lips/teeth.
- **Body of OPA:** Should follow the curve of the tongue, not forcing it backward.
- **Check breathing:**
  - Chest movement with each breath.
  - Airflow felt/seen at mouth and nose.
  - No excessive gagging (if gag reflex appears, remove the OPA).

Correctly Seated OPA

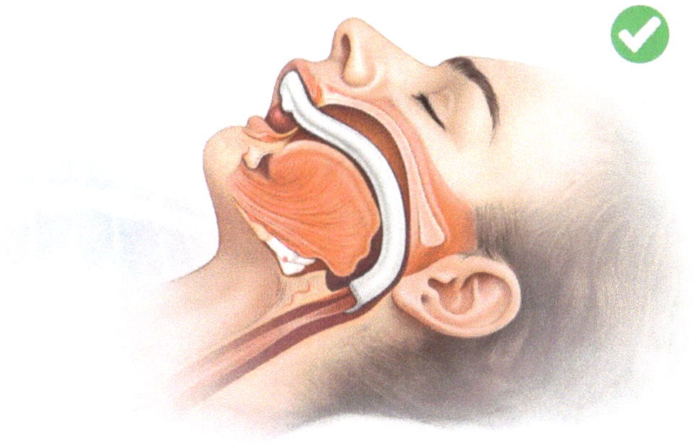

OPA in place, tip resting above the epiglottis in the oropharynx.

Step 7 – Secure and continue care

Text for learners:

- **Stabilise:** Maintain head tilt–chin lift or jaw thrust as indicated.
- **Adjuncts:** Connect to a bag–mask device if providing ventilation.
- **Monitor:** Reassess airway frequently; if the patient regains consciousness or gags, remove the OPA.

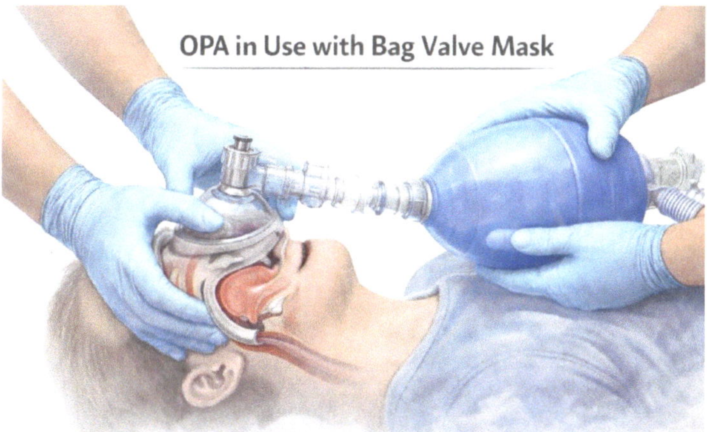

OPA in place, strengthening teamwork and maintaining its airway.

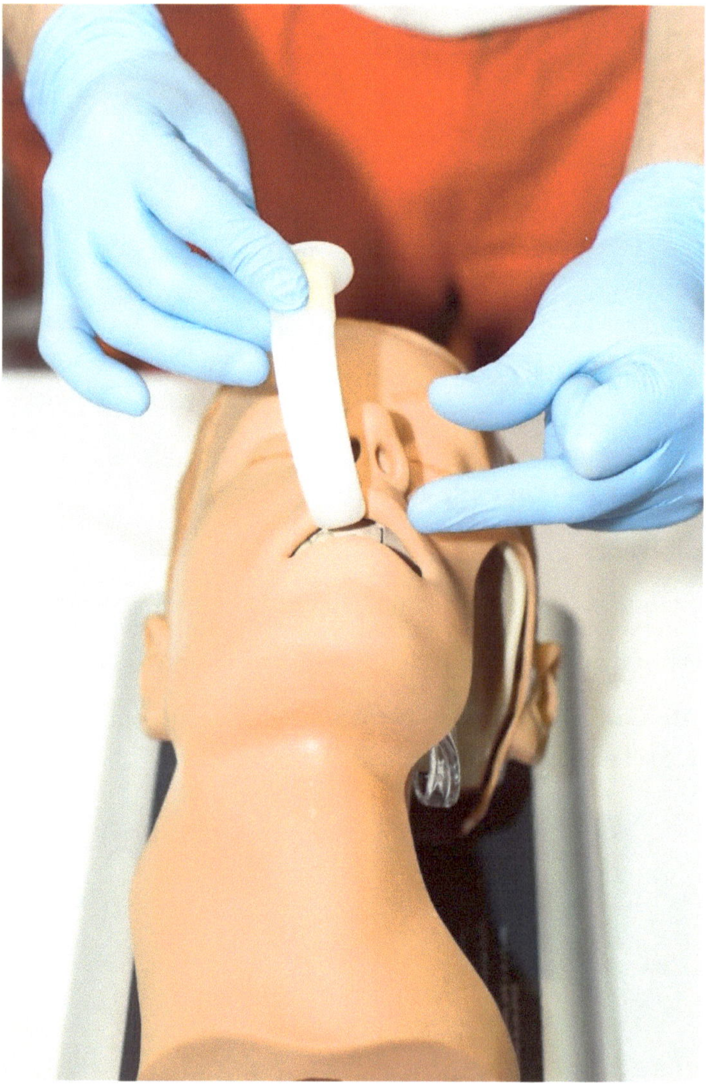

NPA(NASOPHARYNGEAL) AIRWAY

A nasopharyngeal airway (NPA) is a **soft, flexible tube** designed to keep the **upper airway open** by sitting in the nasal passage and extending into the back of the throat (the nasopharynx). It is one of the simplest and most reliable adjuncts for maintaining an airway when a patient cannot do so effectively on their own.

Key Features

- Made of soft rubber or plastic
- Inserted through the **nose**, not the mouth
- Sits in the **nasopharynx** (the space behind the nose and above the throat)
- Has a **flange** at the outer end to prevent it slipping inside
- Comes in varied sizes for adults and children

Why It is Useful in Emergencies

- Easy and quick to insert
- Well tolerated by patients with a gag reflex
- Helps maintain airway patency during seizures, reduced consciousness, or medical collapse
- Can be used alongside oxygen delivery and basic airway manoeuvres

Nasopharyngeal Airway (NPA) Insertion

1. Indications and checks

A. **Confirm need for an NPA**

- **Use an NPA when:**
  - The patient has reduced consciousness but still has a gag reflex.
  - You cannot maintain the airway with simple manoeuvres alone (e.g. jaw thrust, chin lift).
- **Avoid NPA if:**
  - Suspected basal skull fracture (e.g. periorbital bruising, CSF leak from nose/ears).
  - Severe facial trauma or distorted nasal anatomy.

B. **Explain and prepare**

- **If conscious or semi-conscious:** briefly explain what you are doing.
- **Apply standard PPE:** gloves, eye protection if needed.

2. Choose the correct size

3. **Select size using external landmarks**
   - Measure from the **tip of the patient's nose** to the **earlobe** or **angle of the jaw**.
   - The chosen NPA should match this length.
4. **Check diameter**
   - The **outer diameter** should be the size of the patient's smallest nostril.
   - Do not force a tube that is clearly too large.

3. Prepare the device

5. **Inspect the NPA**
   - Check for cracks, deformities, or sharp edges.
   - Ensure the **flange** at the proximal end is intact (prevents the NPA disappearing into the nose).
6. **Lubricate**
   - Apply a **water-based lubricant** generously to the distal (inserted) end.
   - Avoid oil-based lubricants.

4. Position the patient

7. **Optimal position**
   - If possible, position the patient in the **neutral position** (head in line with body).
   - In suspected spinal injury, **do not** use head tilt; maintain manual in-line stabilisation if indicated.

8. **Choose the nostril**

    - Usually insert into the **right nostril first** (often straighter), unless obstructed or injured.
    - If resistance is met, you can try the other nostril with the same or a smaller size.

5. Insert the NPA

9. **Initial orientation**

    - Hold the NPA with the **bevel facing towards the septum** (flat side towards the middle of the nose).

10. **Insertion technique**

- Gently lift the tip of the patient's nose slightly upwards.
- Insert the lubricated tip into the nostril, **directing it along the floor of the nasal cavity**, not upwards.
- Advance with a **gentle, steady twisting or rotating motion**, following the natural curve of the airway.

11. **Do NOT force the tube**

- If you meet firm resistance:
    - Stop.
    - Withdraw slightly.
    - Reassess size and direction or try the **other nostril**.

6. Final positioning and confirmation

12. **Correct depth**

- Advance until the **flange rests comfortably against the nostril**.
- The distal tip should now sit in the **nasopharynx**, just above the oropharynx.

13. **Check effectiveness**

- Look, listen, and feel for **improved airflow**.
- Observe **chest movement** and listen for air entry.

- The patient may tolerate it with minimal gagging or coughing (especially if drowsy).

14. **Secure the airway**

- If needed, use tape or a dressing strip to stabilise the NPA at the nostril (without occluding it).
- Combine with **jaw thrust or chin lift** if required to optimise the airway.

7. Ongoing monitoring

15. **Monitor continuously**

- Reassess **airway, breathing, and consciousness** regularly (DRABCDE).
- Watch for:
    - Increased obstruction noise
    - Bleeding from the nostril
    - Dislodgement or patient intolerance

16. **Remove if necessary**

- If the patient gags persistently, coughs violently, or becomes very distressed, gently remove the NPA.
- Revert to basic airway manoeuvres and reassess.

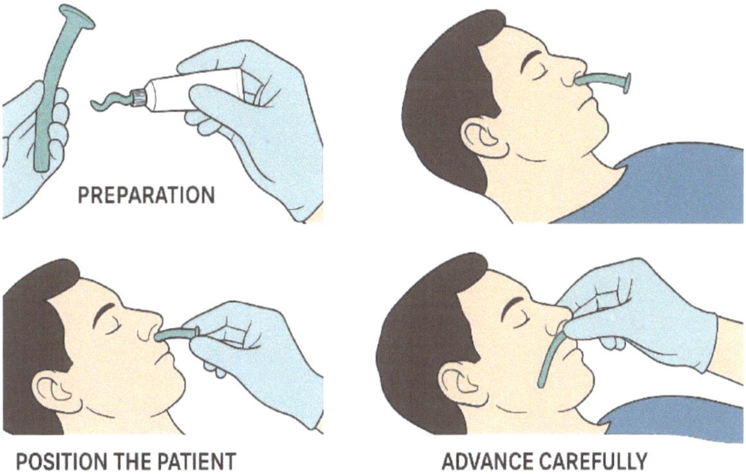

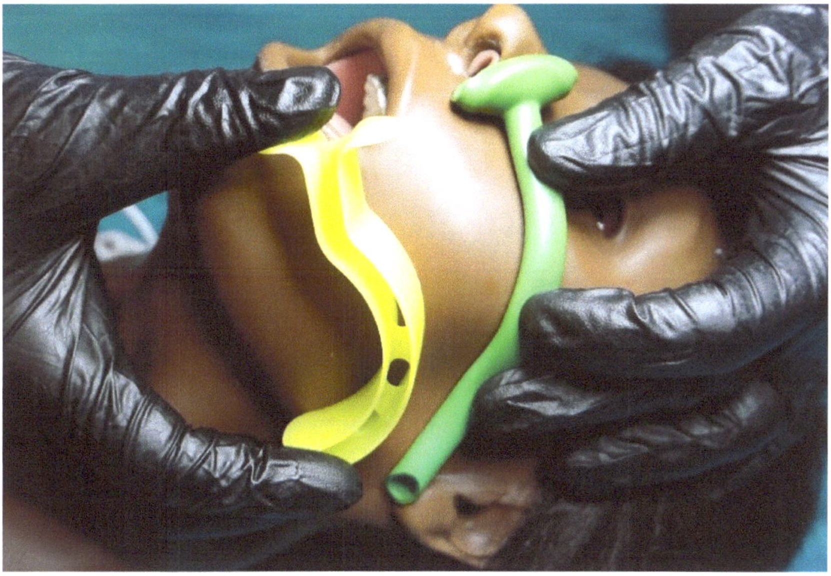

JAW THRUST

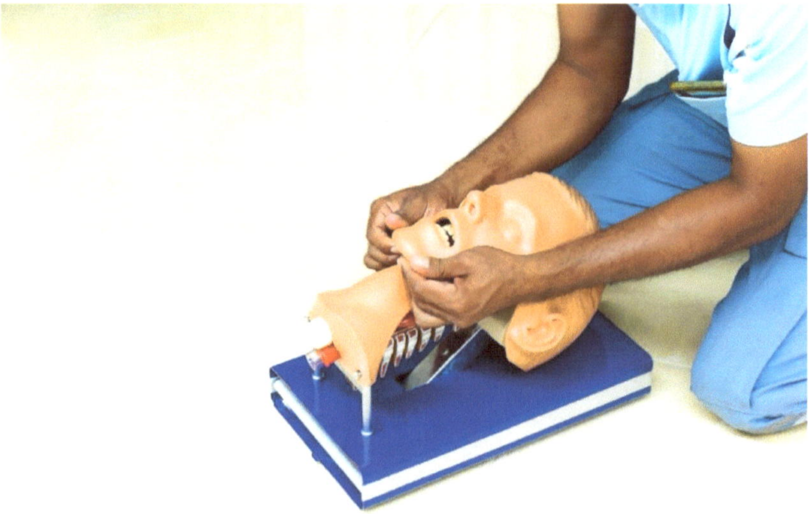

Jaw Thrust Technique (Airway Manoeuvre)

What is the Jaw Thrust?

The **jaw thrust** is a manual airway-opening technique used to **maintain a clear airway without moving the neck**.
It is essential to consider a cervical spine injury when it **is suspected**.

When to Use the Jaw Thrust

Use the jaw thrust when:

- The patient is **unconscious**
- There is **suspected head, neck, or spinal trauma**
- You need to open the airway **without head tilt**
- Managing airway during trauma or immobilisation

How the Jaw Thrust Works

- Lifting the **mandible (lower jaw)** forward

- Moves the **tongue and soft tissues away** from the back of the throat
- Opens the airway while keeping the neck neutral

Step-by-Step Jaw Thrust Technique

1. **Position yourself**
    - Kneel at the **head of the patient**
    - Ensure the head and neck remain **neutral and aligned**
2. **Hand placement**
    - Place your **index and middle fingers** behind the **angles of the mandible** (jawbone)
    - Place your **thumbs** lightly on the chin or lower lip
3. **Apply the thrust**
    - Push the jaw **upward and forward**
    - Lift the mandible toward the ceiling
    - Do **not** tilt the head or flex/extend the neck
4. **Open the mouth (if needed)**
    - Use your thumbs to gently open the mouth
    - Maintain forward jaw pressure

Signs the Jaw Thrust Is Effective

- Improved airflow
- Visible chest rise
- Reduced snoring or gurgling sounds
- Easier ventilation with BVM

Important Points & Safety Tips

- Can be **uncomfortable** in semi-conscious patients
- If the patient **gags, resists, or regains consciousness**, reassess
- Maintain **manual in-line stabilisation** if spinal injury is suspected

- If ineffective, escalate to adjuncts (OPA/NPA if appropriate)

Jaw Thrust vs Head Tilt–Chin Lift

Jaw Thrust	Head Tilt–Chin Lift
No neck movement	Requires neck extension
Used in trauma	Avoid in suspected trauma
More difficult to maintain	Easier for single rescuer

✓ Jaw thrust opens the airway **without moving the neck**

✓ First-line airway manoeuvre in **trauma patients**

✓ Requires correct hand placement and steady forward pressure

HEAD TILT, CHIN LIFT

Head Tilt–Chin Lift Technique (Airway Manoeuvre)

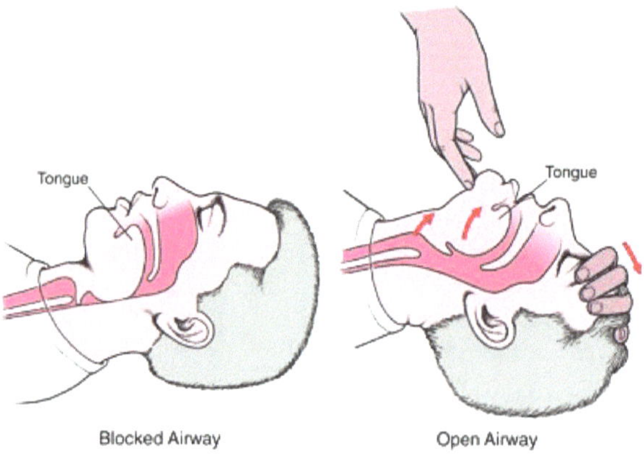

What is the Head Tilt–Chin Lift?

The **head tilt–chin lift** is a **basic airway-opening technique** used to open the airway in an **unconscious patient** by lifting the tongue away from the back of the throat.

It is the **first-line airway manoeuvre** when **NO spinal injury is suspected**.

When to Use Head Tilt–Chin Lift

Use this technique when:

- The patient is **unconscious**
- There is **no suspicion of head, neck, or spinal injury**
- The airway is obstructed by the **tongue**
- You need to improve breathing or assist ventilation

How It Works

- Tilting the head **extends the neck**
- Lifting the chin **pulls the tongue forward**
- This clears the airway and allows air to pass into the lungs

Step-by-Step Technique

1. **Position the patient**
    - Patient lying on their back
    - Kneel beside or at the head
2. **Head tilt**
    - Place one hand on the **forehead**
    - Gently tilt the head **backwards**
3. **Chin lift**
    - Place two fingers under the **bony part of the chin**
    - Lift the chin **upwards and forwards**
4. **Open the mouth**

- Allow the mouth to open naturally
- Do **not** press on the soft tissues under the chin

Signs the Technique Is Effective

- Improved airflow
- Chest rise visible
- Reduced snoring or gurgling sounds
- Easier breathing or ventilation with BVM

When NOT to Use Head Tilt–Chin Lift

Do **not** use if:

- **Spinal injury is suspected**
- Patient has significant **head or neck trauma**

→ Use a **jaw thrust** instead in these situations.

Common Errors to Avoid

- Pressing on the soft tissue under the chin (can block the airway)
- Insufficient head tilt
- Using the technique on a patient with suspected spinal injury

Head Tilt–Chin Lift vs Jaw Thrust

Head Tilt–Chin Lift	Jaw Thrust
Requires neck movement	No neck movement
Non-trauma patients	Suspected trauma
Easier to perform	More difficult, but safer in trauma

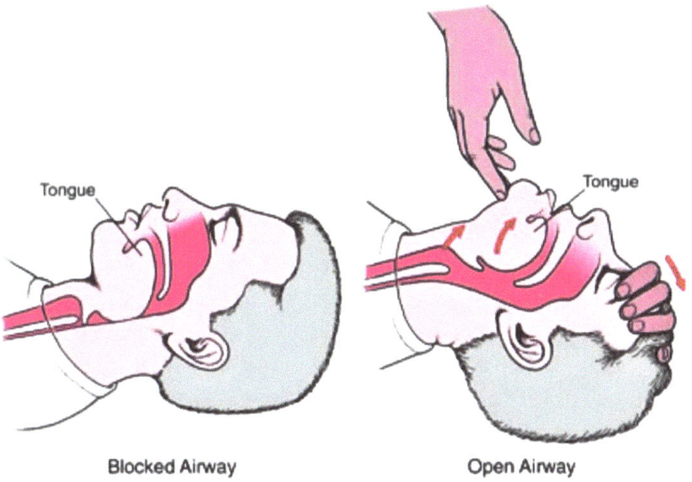

CARDIOPULMONARY RESUSCITATION (CPR)

Core Principles of CPR (All Ages)

- Ensure the **safety** of the rescuer and the casualty
- **Early recognition** of cardiac arrest
- **Early CPR**
- **Early defibrillation**
- **Early advanced care**

If unresponsive and not breathing normally → start CPR immediately and send for a defibrillator.

ADULT CPR

Ensure the scene is safe for you and the casualty.

CHECK IF THE PATIENT IS RESPONSIVE

Kneel beside him.

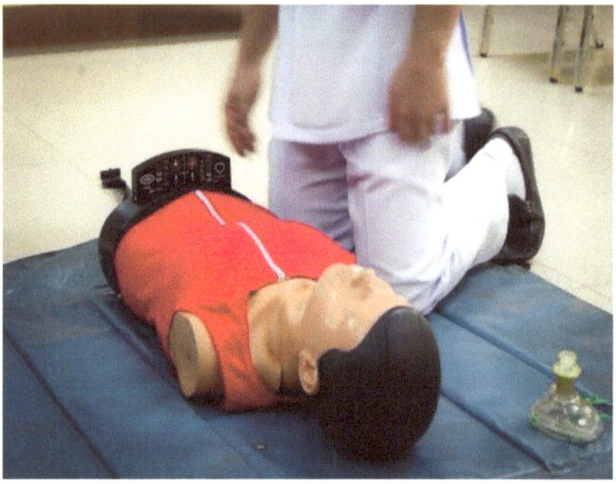

SHAKE THE PATIENT'S SHOULDER OR SQUEEZE THE EARLOBES OR THE TRAPEZIUS MUSCLES

Check whether the casualty is responsive by shaking the casualty's shoulder, speaking to the casualty, and saying, "Wake up!" "Squeeze my hand, squeeze the ear lobes, or press the supraorbital notch or the trapezius

muscle.

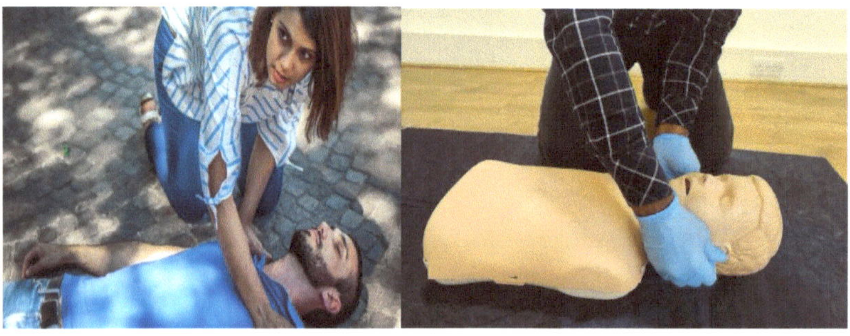

CALL 999/112 OR ASK A BYSTANDER TO CALL IF THE PATIENT IS UNRESPONSIVE. CALL 2222 IF IN THE HOSPITAL.

If unresponsive, proceed immediately to emergency call. Call first before checking breathing; call handlers will assist with breathing assessment.

- Ask for an **ambulance and AED**.
- If alone, use a hands-free speaker or phone headset.
- Dispatchers will help assess and guide CPR.

Give your location, your name, the names of the casualty, and the patient's condition. Ask for oxygen, a defibrillator, and any other resources you require to assist you in conducting adequate resuscitation.

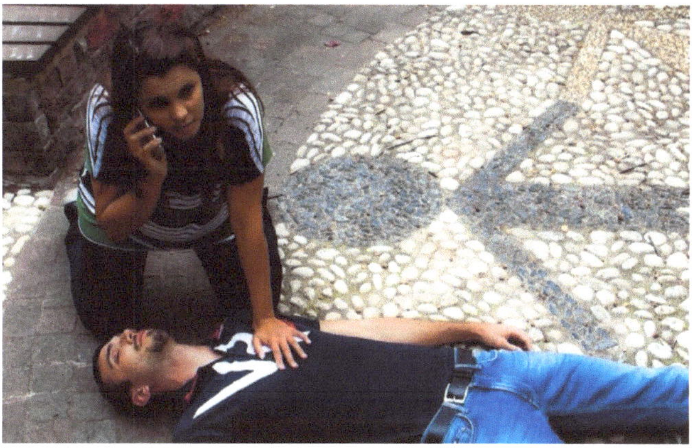

Place one hand on the forehead.

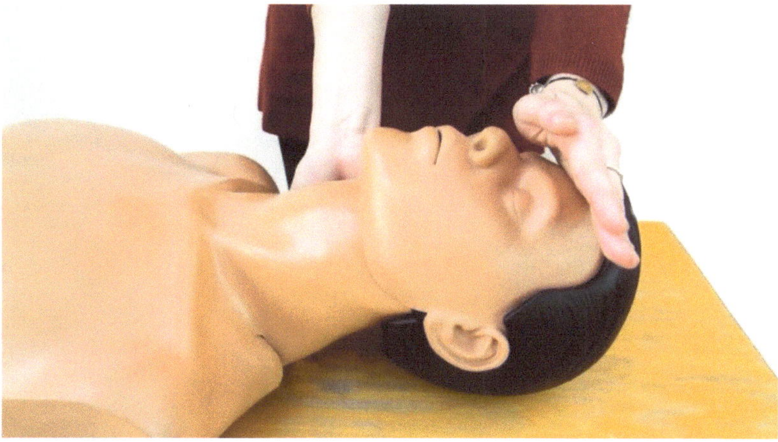

DO A HEAD TILT, CHIN LIFT

To maintain a clear airway, do a head tilt and chin lift. This will elevate the patient's relaxed tongue from the back of the airway to the front of the mouth. To achieve this, place your hand on your forehead, then lift your chin with the other hand.

ASSESS BREATHING

- Lower your head close to the casualty's face with your cheek close to the nose so that you can listen for any breath from the casualty's nose, feel the air from the casualty's nose on your cheek, and see the casualty's chest rise and fall. Do this for no more than 10 seconds. If the Casualty is **not breathing normally**, or breathing is **abnormal (agonal gasps)** assume cardiac arrest.
- **Do NOT delay CPR by over-analysing breathing patterns**.

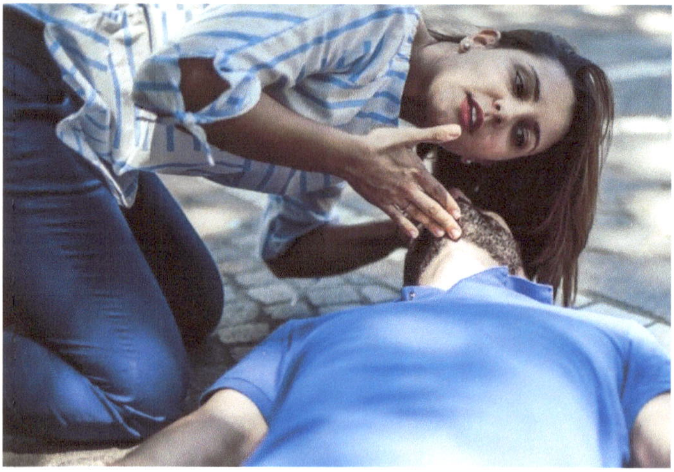

Start CPR Immediately

Chest Compressions

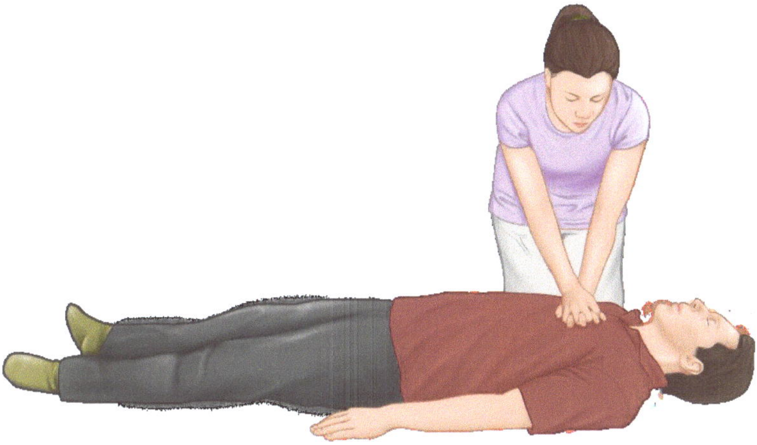

- Hand position: **centre of chest**
- Interlock fingers
- Arms straight, shoulders over hands
- Depth: **5–6 cm**
- Rate: **100–120 per minute**
- Allow **full chest recoil**

Compression–Ventilation Ratio

Conduct chest compressions immediately. For an adult, the ratio of compressions to breath should be thirty to two rescue breaths at 100-120 compressions per minute. On average, you are giving two compressions per second.

- **30 compressions : 2 breaths**

Minimise interruptions

Continue until professional help arrives or AED prompts otherwise.

- Place the heel of your hand in the centre of the patient's Chest slightly above the tip of the breastbone. The position of your hand on the chest is vital to effective CPR.

- Place the second hand on top of the first hand, which is already positioned on the chest. Interlock your fingers and give 30 compressions at a rate of 2 per second.
- 100-120 compressions per minute. Make sure your arms are straight and that you are leaning slightly over the patient.
- Press down on the casualty's chest to a depth of 5-6cm.
- Release your pressure on the chest and watch it recoil before pressing down on the chest again.

Rescue breaths

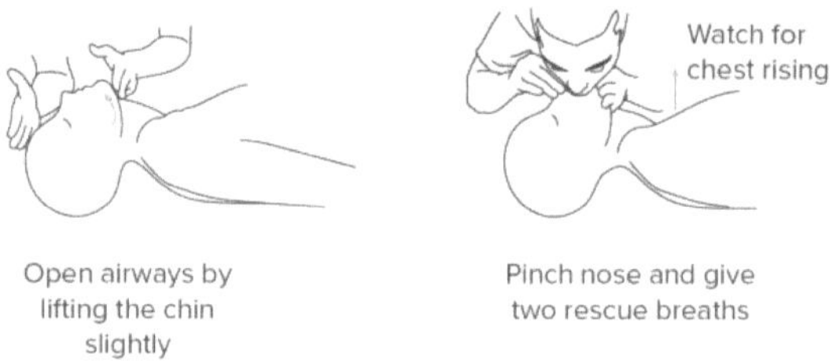

Rescue Breaths

- **If trained and willing**:
  30 compressions: 2 breaths.
- If trained and willing, provide rescue breaths using a barrier device where available. Compression-only CPR is acceptable if unwilling or unable.

Rescue Breath-Mouth-to-Mouth.

Seal your mouth over the patient's mouth whilst squeezing the patient's nose with your left index finger and thumb. Ensure the patient's head is tilted back to clear the airway. Direct mouth-to-mouth should only be attempted if you are sure the patient has no infection, or if you are confident you have no infection that you will pass to the patient. If you have any doubt, conduct compression-only CPR on the patient. Give two rescue breaths to the patient. Each breath should take no more than a second. If unwilling or unable to give breaths → **compression-only CPR**

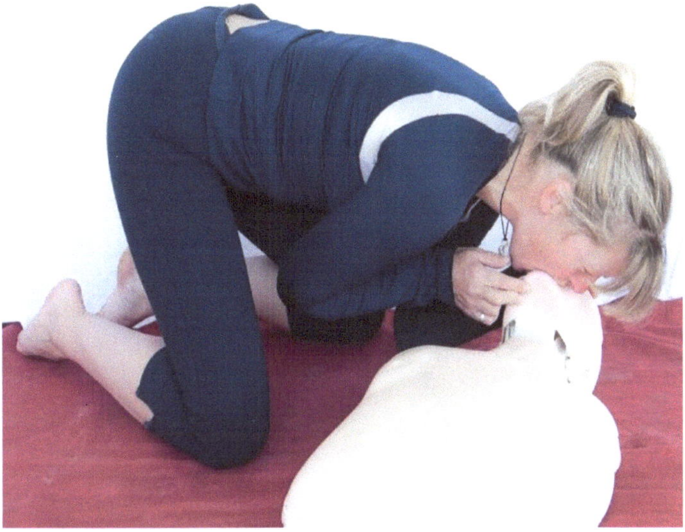

Rescue Breath-Mouth to face shield.

If you have a face shield, use it to minimise the risk of infection for you or the patient.

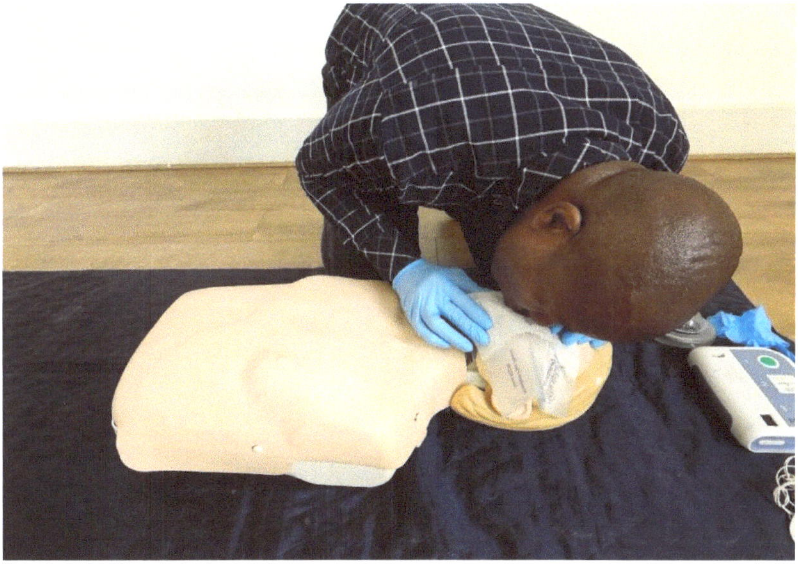

Rescue Breath- Mouth-to-Pocket Mask

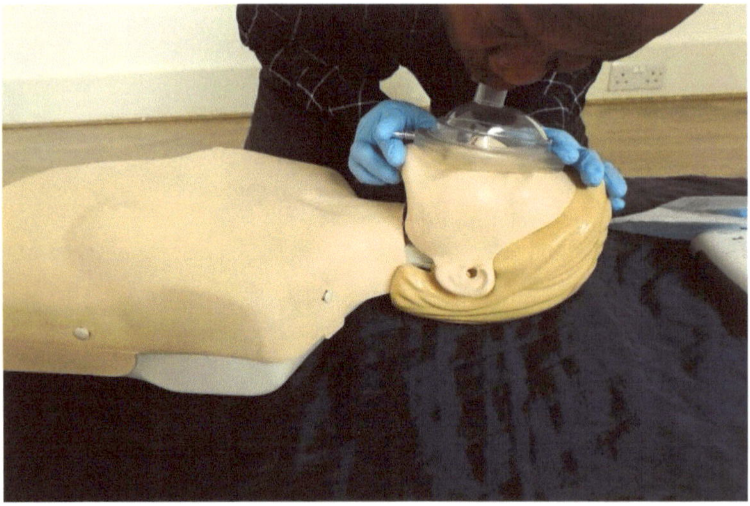

Rescue breathing can also be administered through a pocket Mask. This is another way of minimising the risk of infection.

Rescue Breath

Mouth-to-Bag Valve Mask (One-Person Technique)

Another method of administering rescue breathing is the bag-valve mask (BVM). The BVM can be administered by an individual helper or by two helpers. The techniques are slightly different. When administered by one helper, the helper forms a C-shape over the mask and then squeezes the bag to deliver oxygen to the patient, while the other hand forms an E-shape by tilting the head back.

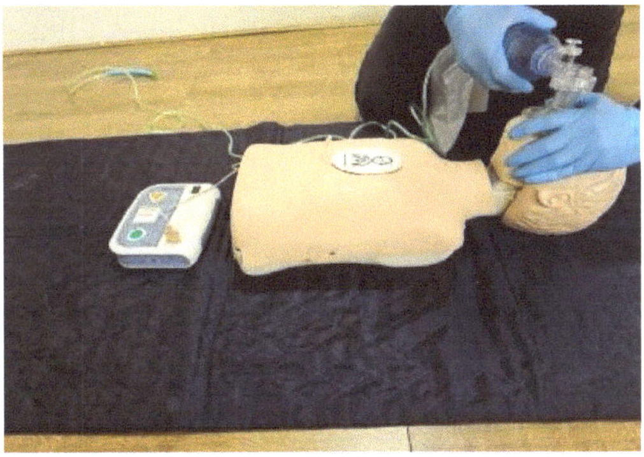

Mouth-to-Bag Valve Mask—Two Persons Technique.

With both hands, one helper seals the BVM mask over the patient's nose and mouth while the other helper presses the oxygen bag to release the oxygen.

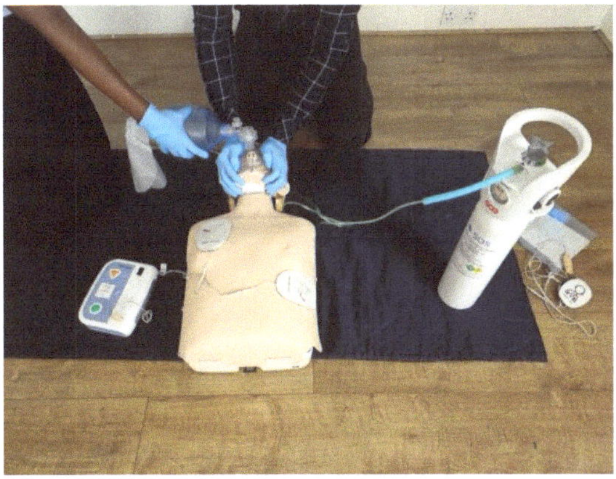

5) Use an AED (Automated External Defibrillator)

1. **Turn on AED as soon as available**
2. **Attach pads** to bare chest as shown on the pads
    - One pad on the **upper right chest**
    - One pad on the **left side below the armpit** (mid-axillary line)
3. Follow **voice prompts**.
4. **Deliver shock if advised**, then **resume CPR immediately**.
5. If repeated shocks are unsuccessful and VF/pVT persists, consider pad repositioning if trained, without delaying CPR.

6) Continue High-Quality CPR

- Continue CPR and AED cycles until:
    - **Signs of life return** (movement, normal breathing),
    - **Advanced responders take over**,
    - Or **you are unable to continue** due to exhaustion.

Special Considerations

If the arrest is due to drowning

→ Give **5 initial rescue breaths** before starting compressions, as hypoxia is the primary cause of arrest in these cases.

Vomiting or airway obstruction

✓ Ensure airway is clear

✓ Continue CPR with breaths if trained

SPECIAL SITUATION: CPR IN LATE PREGNANCY

When performing CPR on a heavily pregnant woman, raise the right hip slightly so that the pregnant woman is leaning slightly to the left side. This shifts the uterus away from the blood vessel, providing an uninterrupted blood supply to the heart.

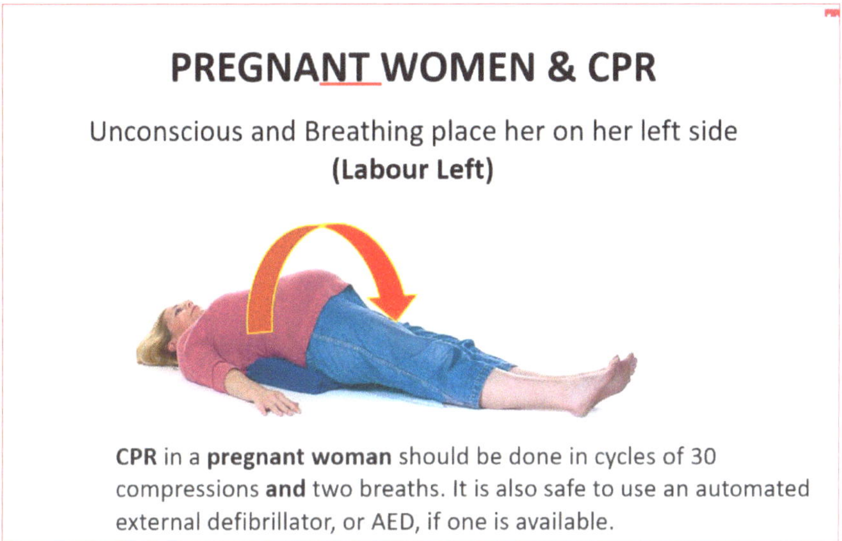

CHILD CPR (1-12)

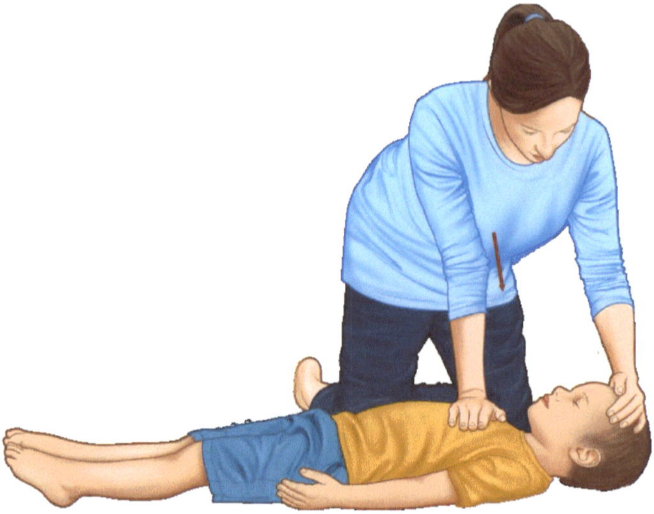

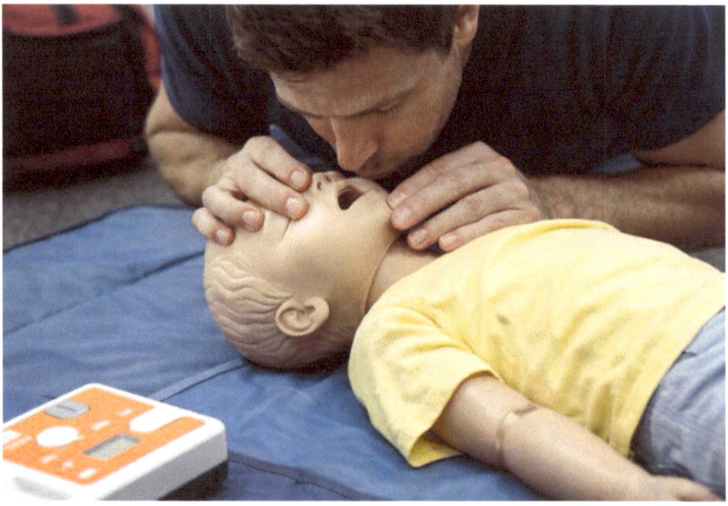

Key Differences

- Cardiac arrest is often **hypoxic**
- Rescue breaths are critical

Sequence

1. Danger

2. Response
3. Airway
4. Breathing
5. **5 initial rescue breaths**

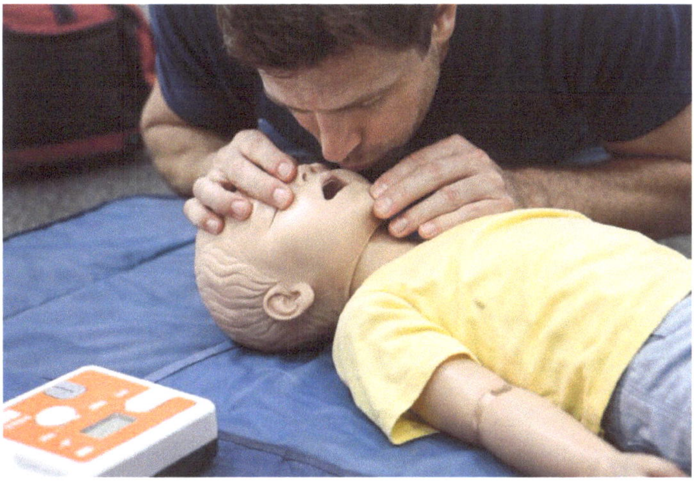

Chest Compressions

- One hand (or two for a larger child)
- Centre of chest
- Depth: **⅓ of chest**
- Rate: **100–120 per minute**

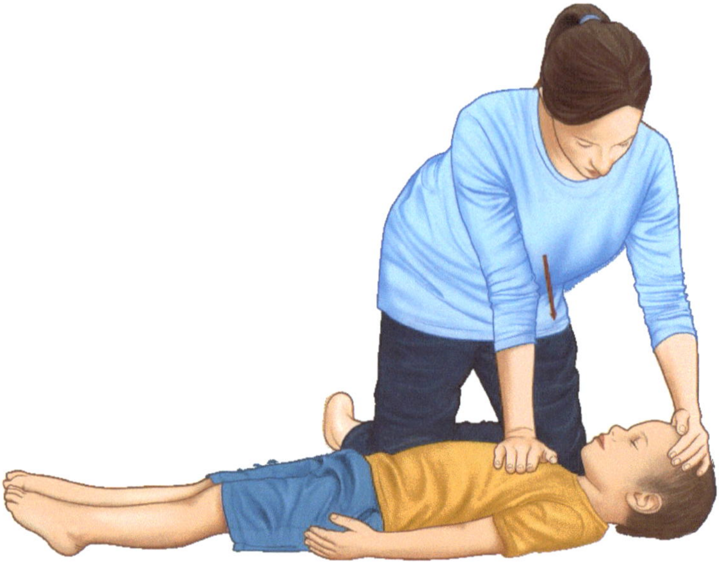

Compression–Ventilation Ratios

- **Healthcare professionals with paediatric duty:**
  15 compressions: 2 breaths
- **Bystanders & most clinicians:**
  30 compressions: 2 breaths

Defibrillation

- Use AED immediately
- Use **paediatric pads** if available
- If pads touch → **front-and-back placement**

INFANT CPR (<1 year)

Response

- Tickle feet
- Observe for movement or sound

Call 999 or 112

Airway

- Neutral head position
- **One finger** chin lift only

Breathing

Give **five rescue breaths**

- Mouth-to-mouth

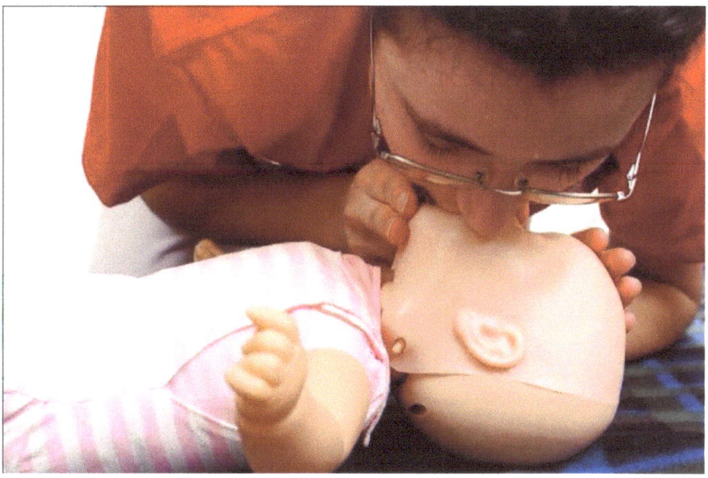

- Or mouth-to-nose if the mouth is injured

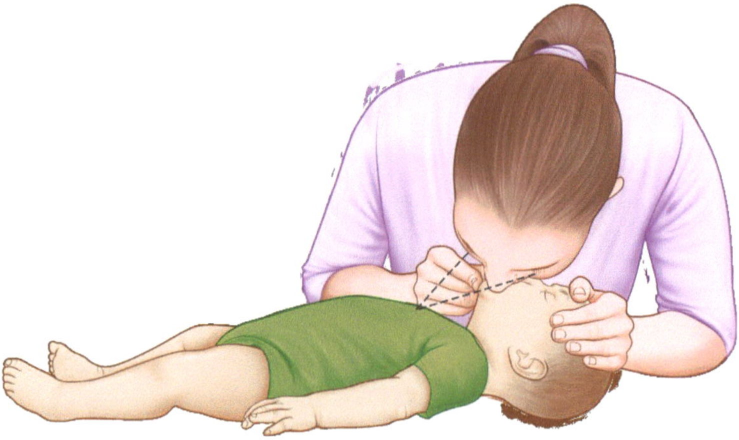

- Mouth to bag valve mask

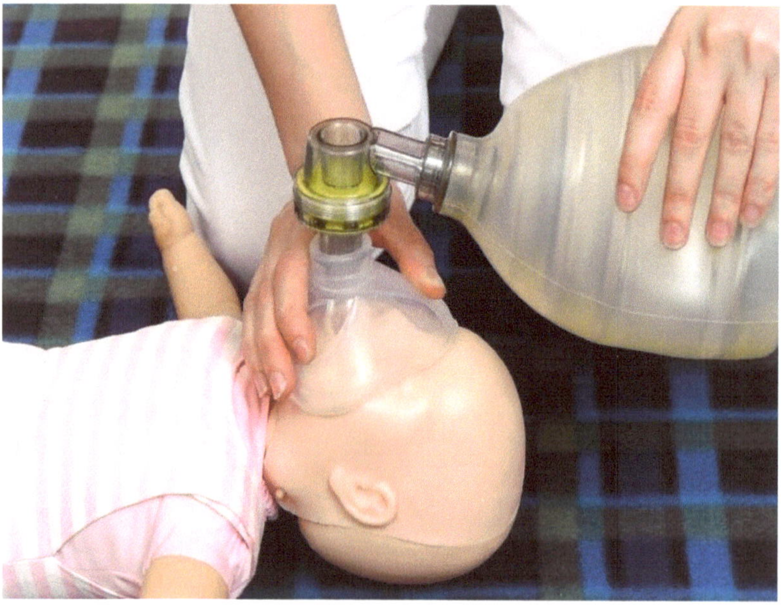

Chest Compressions

- Depth: **⅓ of chest**

Ratios

- **Healthcare professionals with paediatric duty: 15:2**

- **Bystanders:**
  30:2

Defibrillation

- Use an AED as soon as available
- Use paediatric pads if possible
- Pad placement: **front and back.**
- Infant compressions with two thumbs

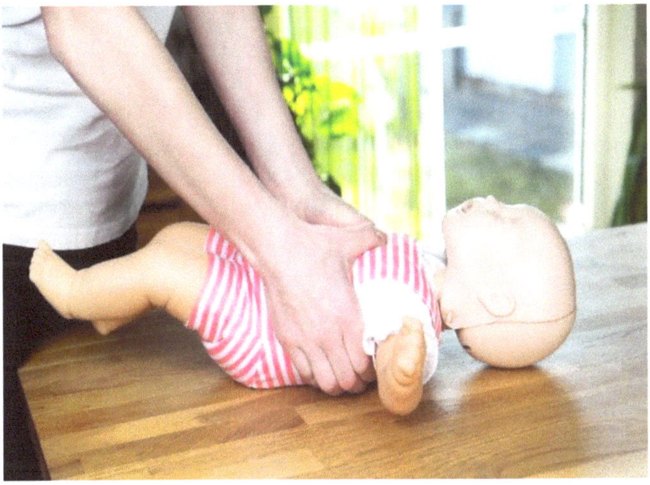

Fig 3. **Chest compression in infants: two-thumb encircling technique**

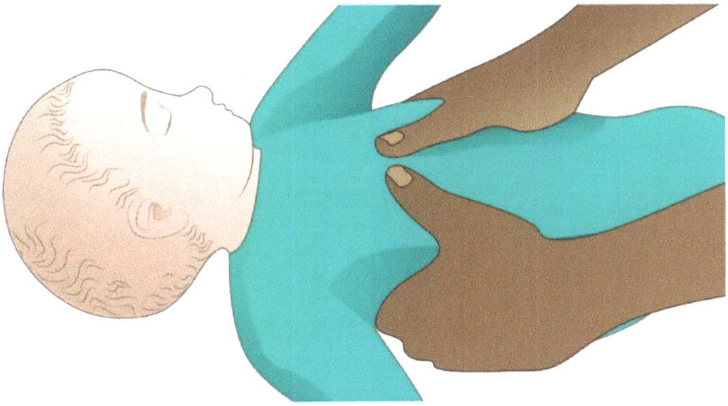

The two-thumb circling technique should be done with the thumbs side by side, and the hands encircling the infant's rib cage

DEFIBRILLATION

Key determinants of successful defibrillation:

- **Time to shock** – earlier defibrillation increases success
- **High-quality CPR** – before and between shocks maintains myocardial perfusion
- **Shockable rhythm** – VF and pulseless VT only
- **Myocardial condition** – oxygenation, perfusion, pH, and electrolytes
- **Correct energy & biphasic waveform**
- **Good pad position & contact** – low transthoracic impedance
- **Underlying cause** – primary cardiac causes respond best

DEFIBRILLATOR SIGNAGE

Every dental practice must have a defibrillator, and staff must know where it is located. The defibrillator signage must be properly displayed and visible to all members of staff and visitors to the practice.

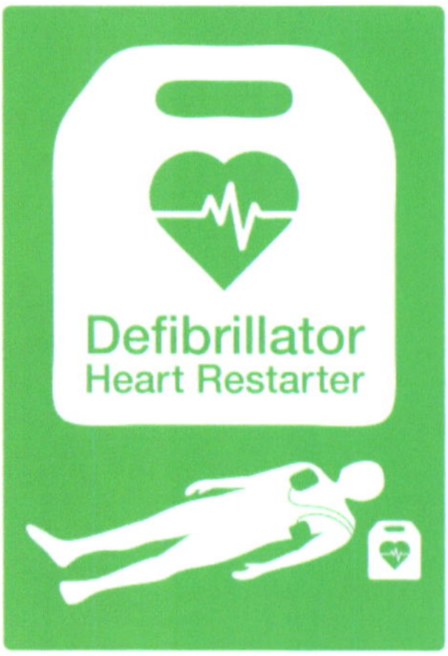

WHAT TO DO WHEN THE AED ARRIVES

Turn the machine on by pushing the on button. For most AEDs, the button will be green.

Making sure the casualty is bare-chested must be the case for all casualties, whether male or female, adult, or child. For female casualties, remove any bra and, if necessary, use scissors to cut through it.

Remove the electrodes or PADS from their seal and remove the backing paper to reveal the sticky part of the pads.

A defibrillator is a device that sends an electric shock to the heart to restore a normal heartbeat.

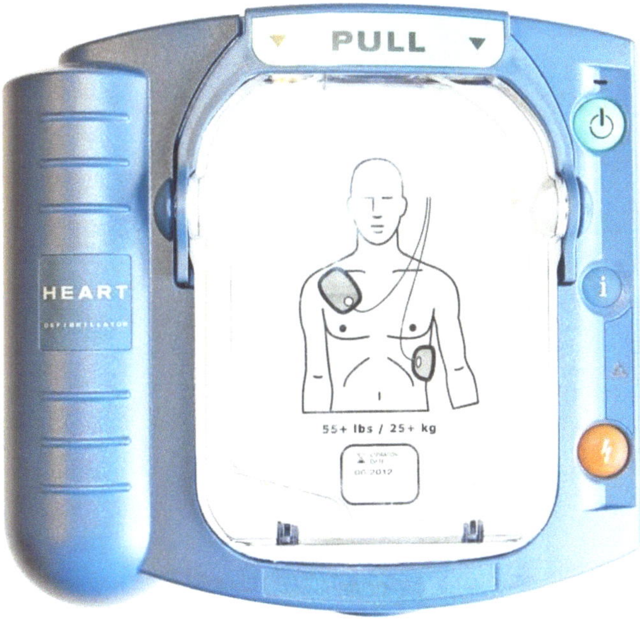

Steps for Using the AED

- When the AED arrives, turn the start button on, and it will automatically begin to issue instructions.
- Attach the electrode pads to the patient's bare chest.
- The AED will begin analysing the patient's heart rhythm. Do not touch the patient while the heart rhythm is being explored.

- If you have a semi-automatic defibrillator, it will ask you to press the shock button to deliver a shock if it detects a shockable rhythm.

Aftershock is delivered, and the AED will instruct you to continue CPR.

Common types of automated external defibrillators.

DEFIBRILLATOR SIGNAGE

Every dental practice must have a defibrillator, and staff must know where it is located. The defibrillator signage must be displayed appropriately and be visible to all staff and visitors to the practice.

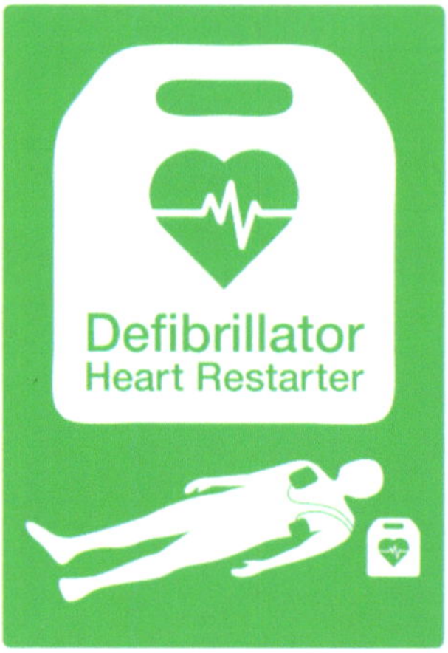

ANTERO-LATERAL PAD PLACEMENT

AED Pad Placement (Adults – Anterior–Lateral Position)

Sternal (Anterior) Pad

- Place one pad on the **right upper chest**
- Position it **just below the right clavicle**
- Ensure it is **to the right of the sternum**

Apical (Lateral) Pad

- Place the second pad on the **left side of the chest**
- Position it **below the left armpit (axilla)**
- Align it along the **mid-axillary line**, level with the nipple (V5–V6 area)

Rationale for This Pad Position

- Creates a **transthoracic electrical pathway** that passes directly through the heart
- **Maximises the likelihood of successful defibrillation**
- Prevents **pad overlap**
- Keeps pads clear of:
    - Excess breast tissue
    - Large muscle groups
    - Implanted devices (where possible)

Key Clinical Notes

- Ensure the chest is **bare, dry, and free of excessive hair** (shave if necessary)
- If a pacemaker or ICD is present, place pads **at least 8 cm away**
- Do **not delay defibrillation** if ideal positioning is not immediately possible

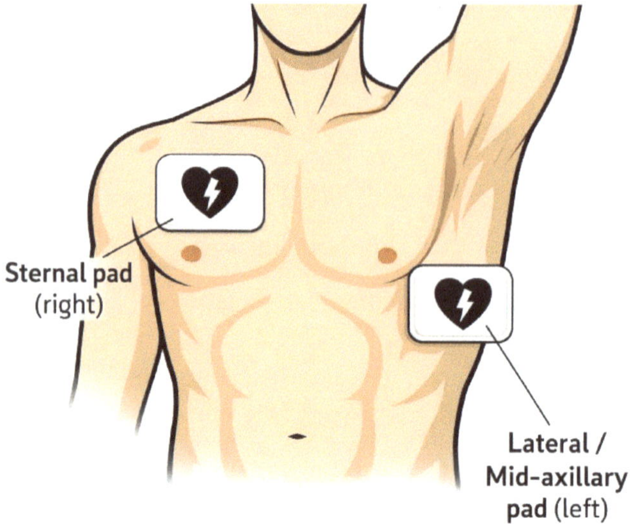
Sternal pad
(right)
Lateral /
Mid-axillary
pad (left)

ANTERIOR-POSTERIOR (AP) AED PAD PLACEMENTS

ANTERIOR (FRONT) PAD

One adhesive pad is placed on the left side of the chest, over the precordium (the cardiac area), just below the left clavicle and lateral to the sternum, over the cardiac apex area.

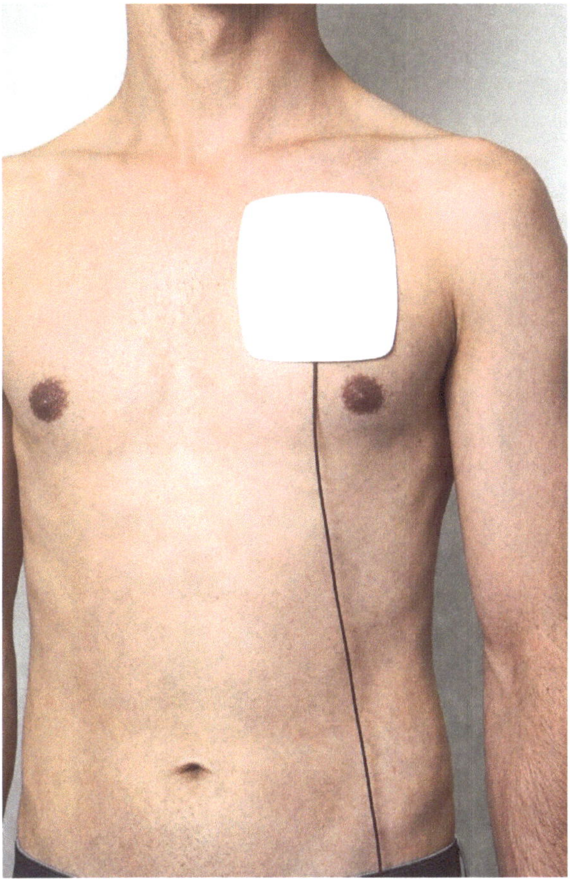

POSTERIOR (BACK) PAD:

The second pad is placed on the back, on the left posterior thorax, below the left scapula and lateral to the spine, at the same horizontal level as the front pad.

The pads are positioned so that the electrical current passes from the front of the chest, traversing the heart,

The anterior-posterior position is commonly used when the anterior–lateral placement is not suitable (e.g., the presence of chest devices, small chest size, or clinical preference).

The placement ensures effective defibrillation by directing current through the myocardium.

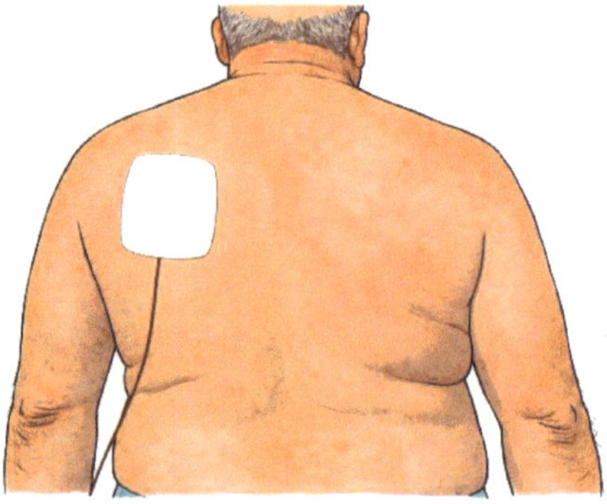

CHILD CPR- DEFIBRILLATING A CHILD- FRONT AND BACK PAD PLACEMENT.

1-12 years Front-Back

- Place the pads in the centre of the chest
- Position it between the nipples
- Back (posterior) pad
- Place on the centre of the back
- Position it between the shoulder blades

The goal is to have one pad on the chest and one on the back, with the heart between them.

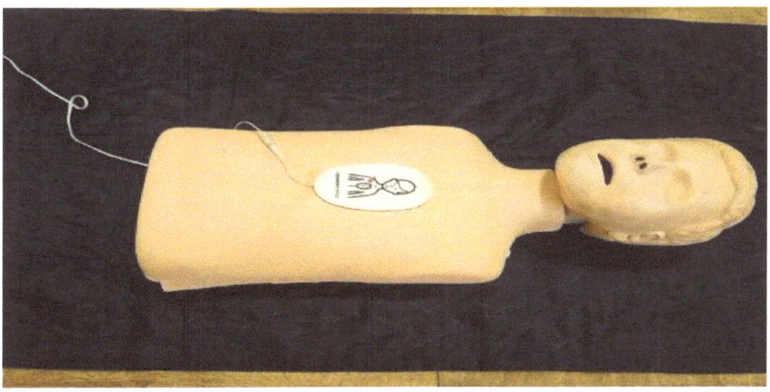

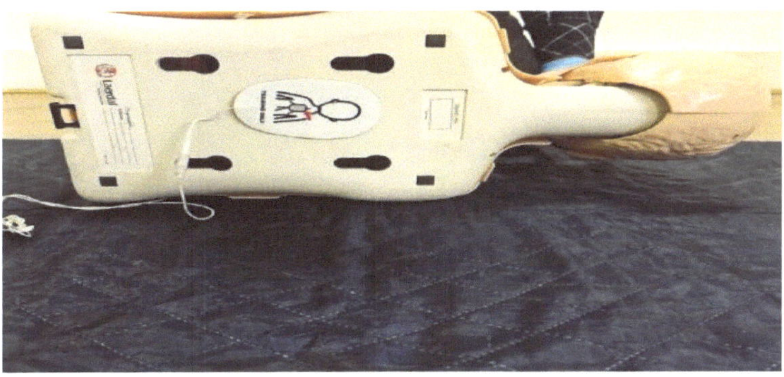

CHILD 13-18 YEARS – (ADOLESCENT) SAME AS ADULT

One pad on the upper right chest, and the other on the left side of the chest under the armpit.

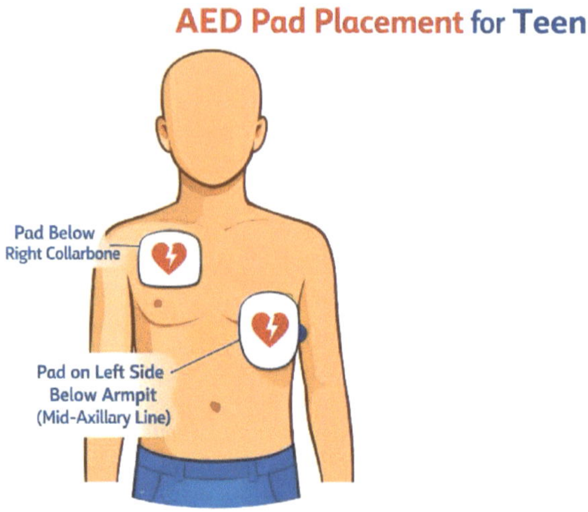

HOW THE AED WORKS

- The pads have sensors called electrodes. When attached to the patient's chest, it sends information about the patient's heart rhythm to the AED's computer. The computer analyses the heart's rhythm to confirm whether a shock is necessary and, if required, will send a shock to correct the abnormal heart rhythm

TYPES OF DEFIBRILLATORS

- Automated External Defibrillators (AEDs)
- Implantable Cardioverter Defibrillators (ICDs)- surgically placed inside the body.
- Wearable Cardioverter Defibrillators (WCDs)-this rests on the body

SAFETY CONSIDERATIONS

JEWELLERY- remove pieces of jewellery and avoid placing the pads on them

MEDICATIONS- Do not place the pads on the pacemaker.

//**CLOTHING**- The patient must be bare-chested.

WATER/SWEAT-wipe any water

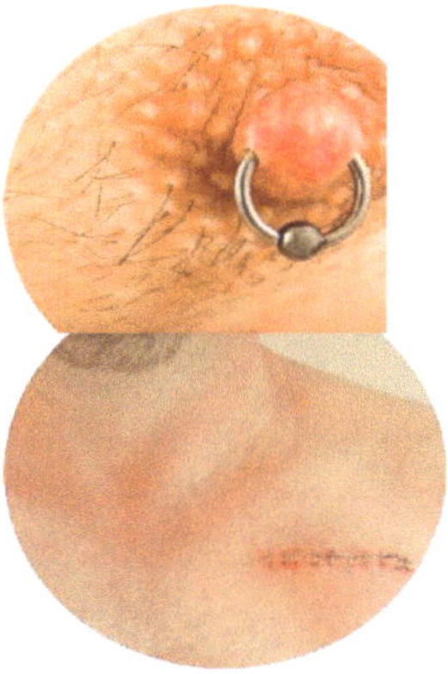

MEDICATIONS do not place pads on the GTN patch.

RESCUE BREATH METHODS (All Ages)

- Mouth-to-mouth
- Mouth-to-mask (preferred)
- Bag-Valve-Mask (BVM)
    - One-person: **C-E grip**
    - Two-person: One seals the mask, one squeezes the bag
- Mouth-to-nose (facial trauma)
- Mouth-to-stoma or tracheostomy (ventilate directly via stoma)

WHEN TO USE 15:2 IN CHILDREN

15:2

- Paediatric doctors & nurses
- Paramedics

- Emergency department staff

30:2

- Members of the public
- Dentists, GPs, school nurses
- Lone responders

Rationale: Simplicity and likelihood of adult CPR scenarios

RECOVERY POSITION (Breathing but Unresponsive adult)

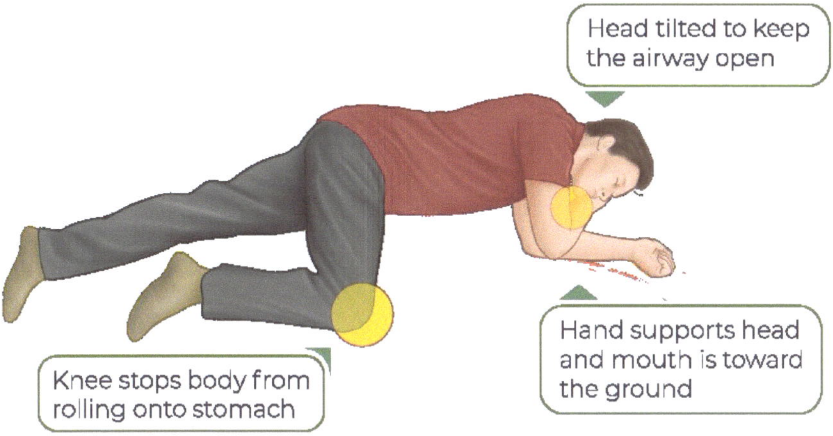

- Place in **lateral position**
- Head tilted, airway open
- Monitor breathing continuously

CHILD RECOVERY POSITION

CHECK FOR DANGER

Make sure you and the patient are safe.

CHECK FOR RESPONSIVENESS

Check whether the patient responds to a painful stimulus by squeezing the earlobes.

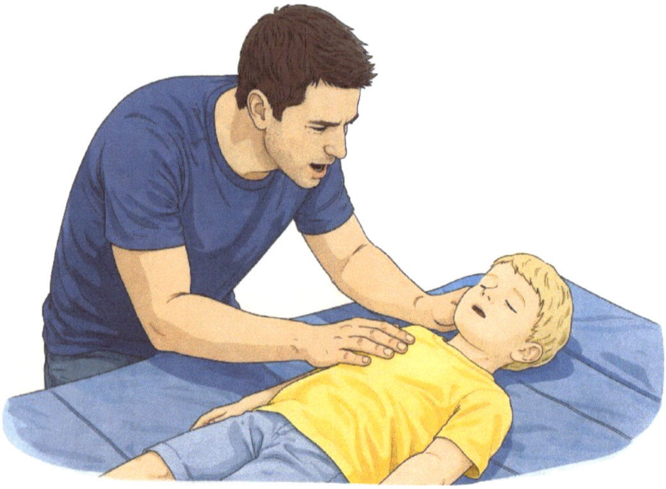

CHILD HEAD TILT, CHIN LIFT

Place one hand on the forehead and two fingers on the chin, tilt your head, and lift your chin.

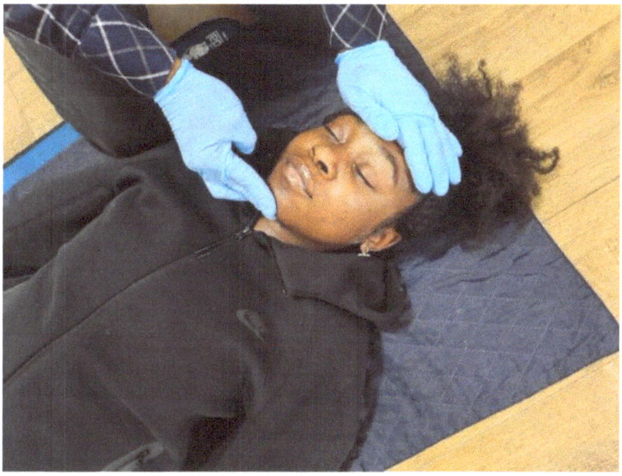

CHECK IF THE CHILD IS BREATHING

Lean towards the head with your cheek facing the casualty's nose to feel for the child's breath.

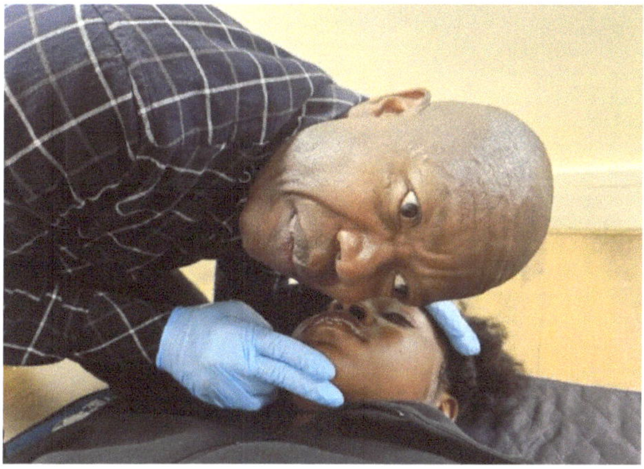

Reach for the casualty's hand nearest you and put it in an angled Or straight position.

Reach out for The Casualty's Hand further from you. Place it on their Cheek And Hold It there.

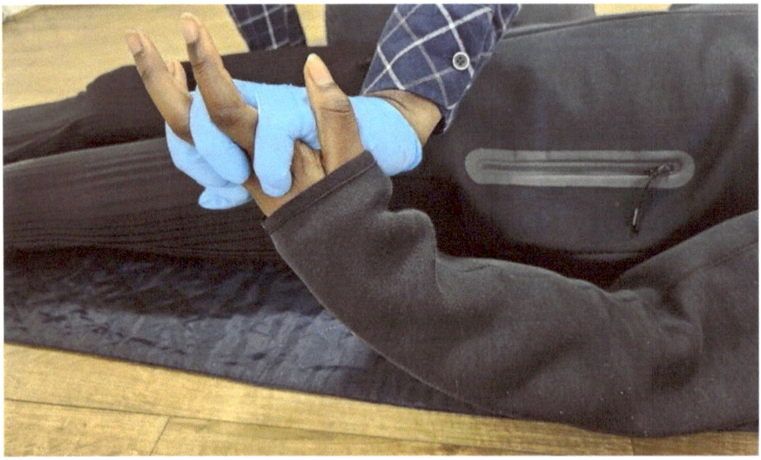

Place the back of the child's hand on their cheek and hold it palm to palm.

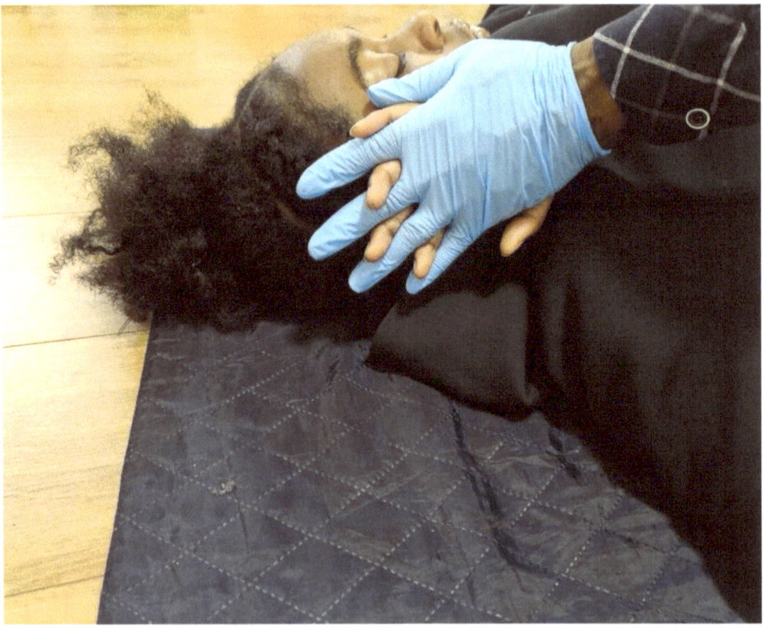

Check the patient's pockets for any sharp objects that could harm the patient.

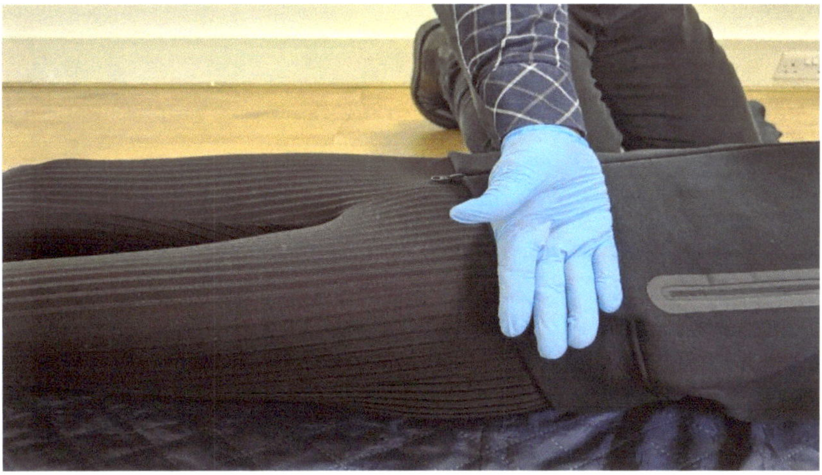

Check the pockets for Sharp objects that can harm the child when you are on her side.

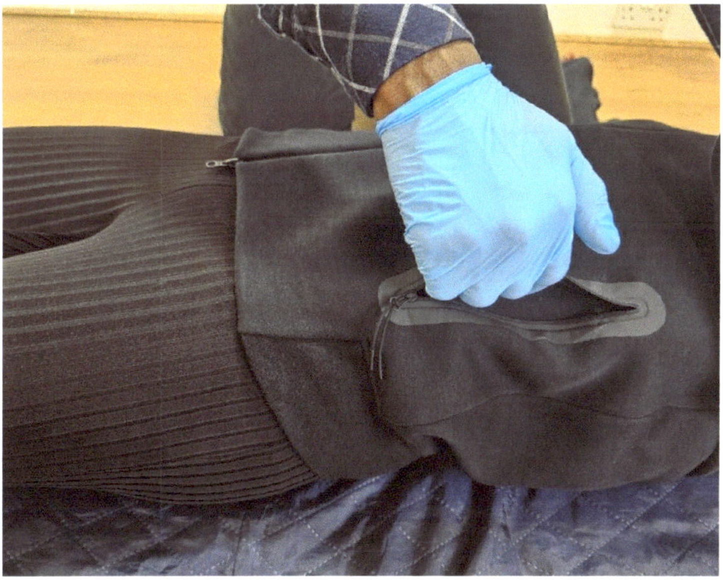

Place your hand on the outer part of the child's leg, which is furthest from you, around the knee.

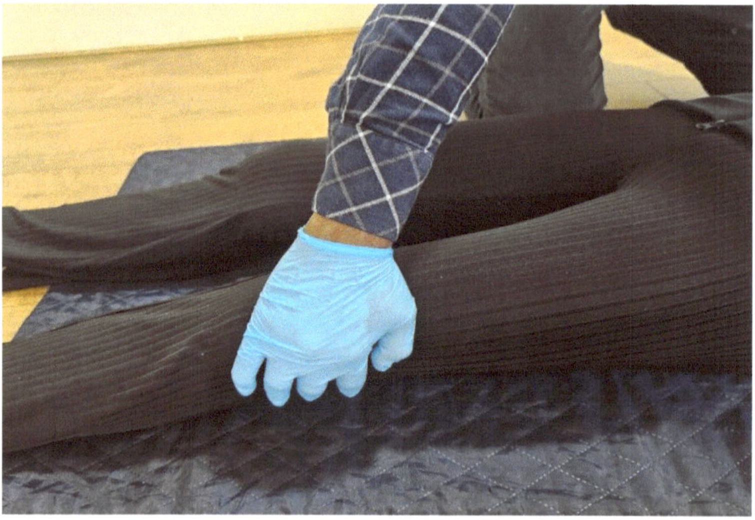

Reach for the leg farther from you and raise it from the Outer part of the knee area, Making Sure the feet are firmly on the ground. Then, lean the casualty towards you.

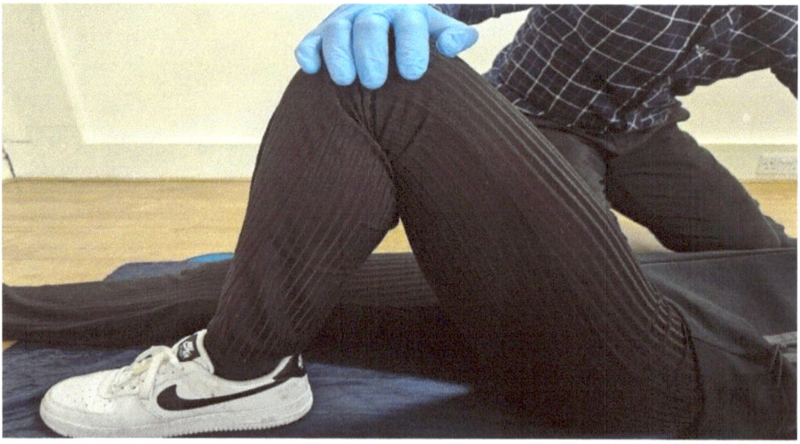

Lift the leg with your hand on the child's knee. Using the knee as a lever, roll the child on her side in a recovery position. Tilt the head back carefully to maintain a clear airway. Check every minute to confirm the child is still breathing whilst waiting for an ambulance to arrive.

TILT THE CHIN UP TO CLEAR THE CASUALTY'S AIRWAY

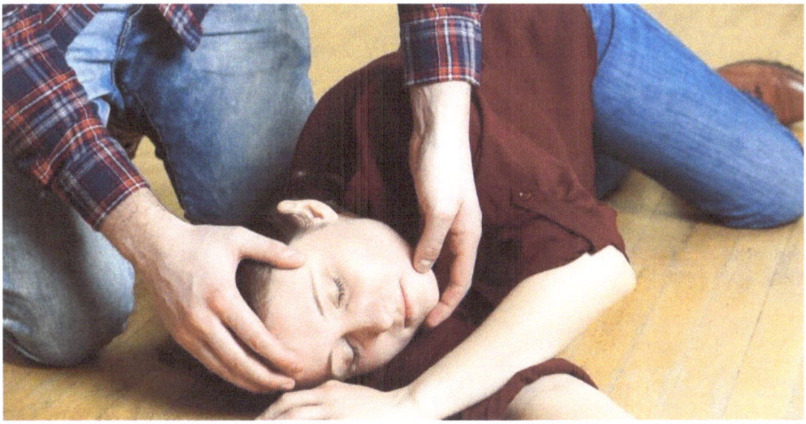

RECOVERY POSITION BABY

CHECK IF BABY IS RESPONSIVE

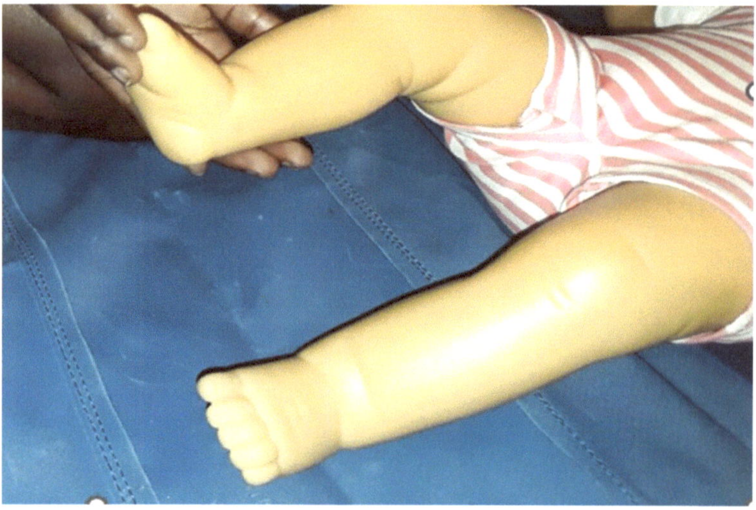

CALL 999/112 IF BABY IS UNRESPONSIVE

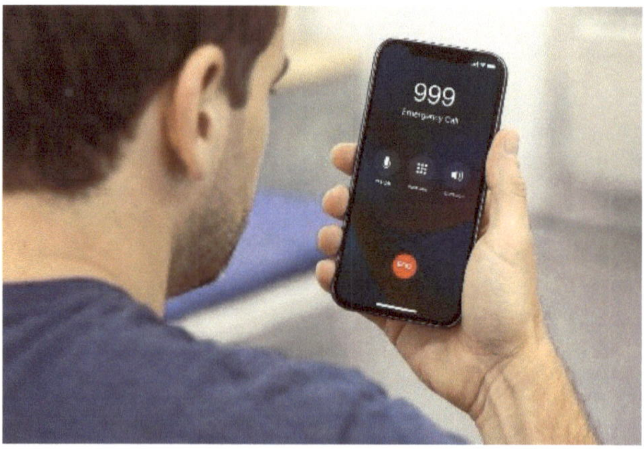

CHECK THE AIRWAY- HEAD TILT AND CHIN LIFT.

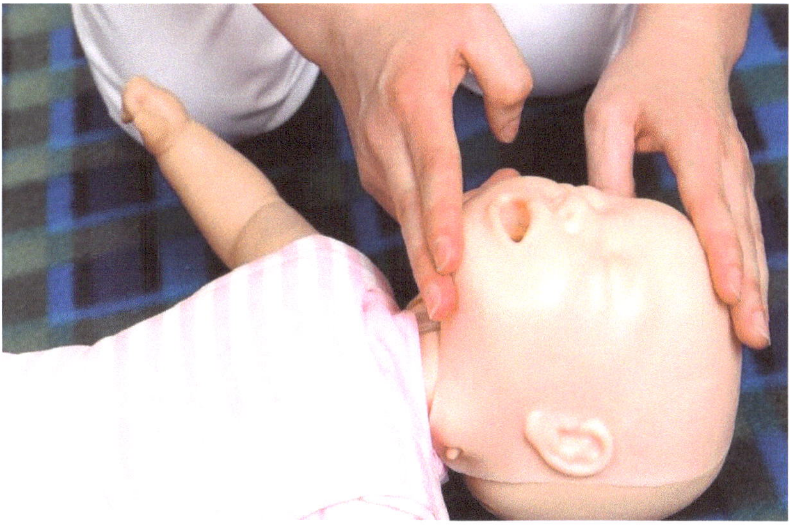

CHECK BREATHING.

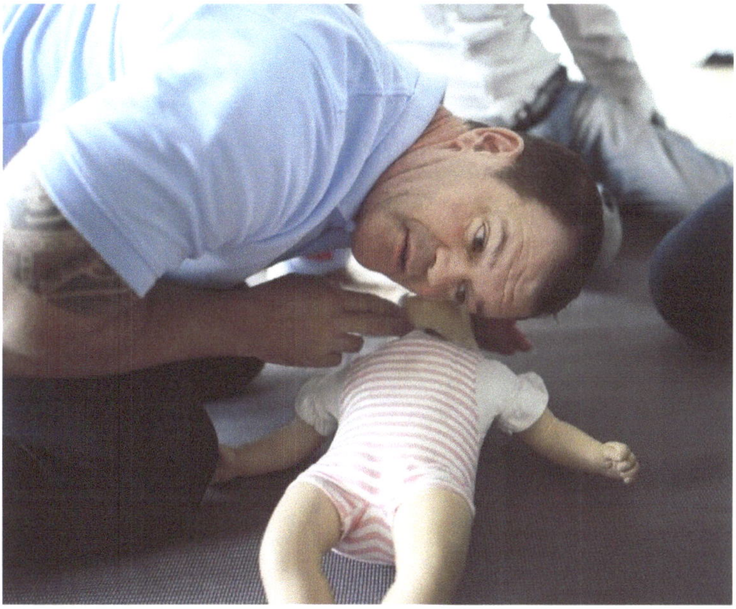

HOLD IN SIDE-LYING OR PRONE POSITION

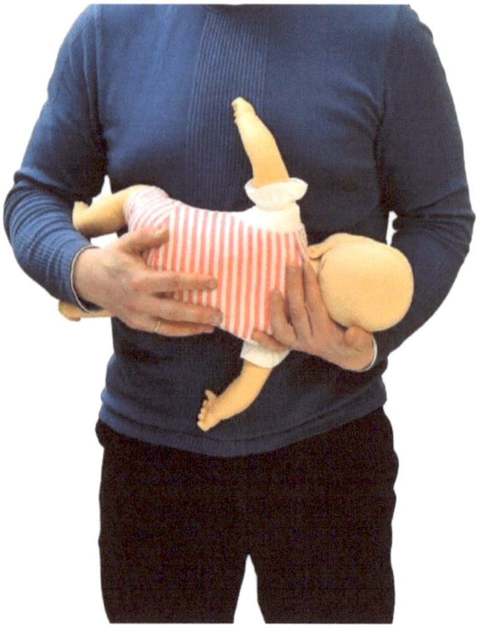

- Head lower than body
- Maintain airway alignment

USING THE AUTOMATED EXTERNAL DEFIBRILLATOR

ADULT CHOKING

WHAT IS CHOKING?

Choking occurs when the airway is partially or fully blocked, preventing air from reaching the lungs. This can happen anywhere from the mouth down to where the windpipe splits into the lungs.

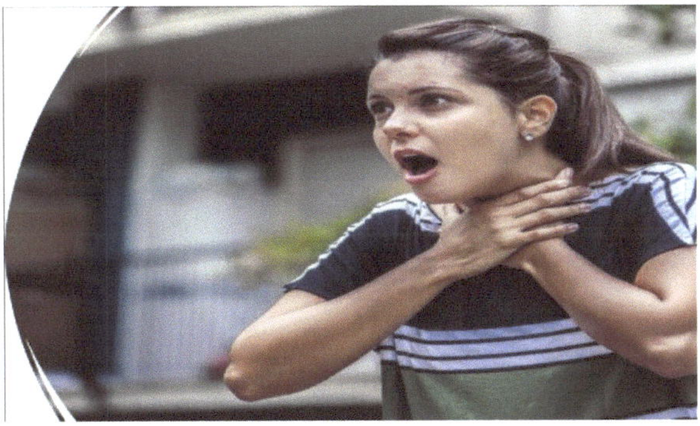

Mild Choking- adult

Mild choking occurs when the airway is only partially blocked, and the patient can still **breathe, cough, or speak**.

- **What to do:**
  - Encourage the patient to **cough forcefully**.
  - Do **not interfere** if they can clear the obstruction themselves.
  - **Do not give back blows or chest thrusts** unless the airway becomes entirely blocked.

Severe Choking

Severe choking usually involves complete airway obstruction. The person will not be able to speak. To help them, you must immediately commence five back Blows followed by five abdominal thrusts. If the treatment does not work, the patient will, at some point, become unconscious and not breathing. It would be best if you commenced CPR immediately.

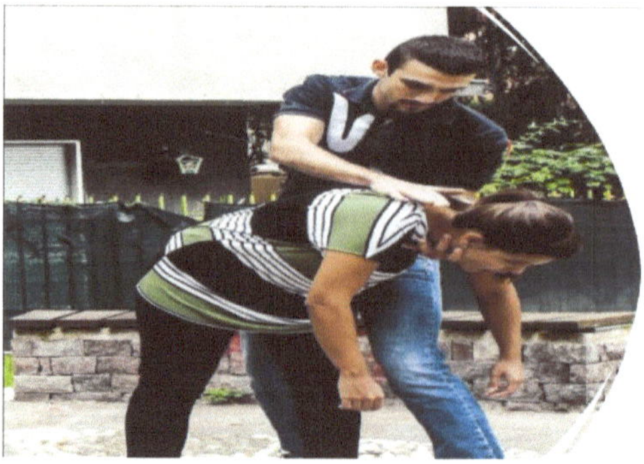

Abdominal thrusts

Make a fist with your dominant hand, and then place that fist above the navel and below the tip of the sternum. Press backwards and upwards up to five times.

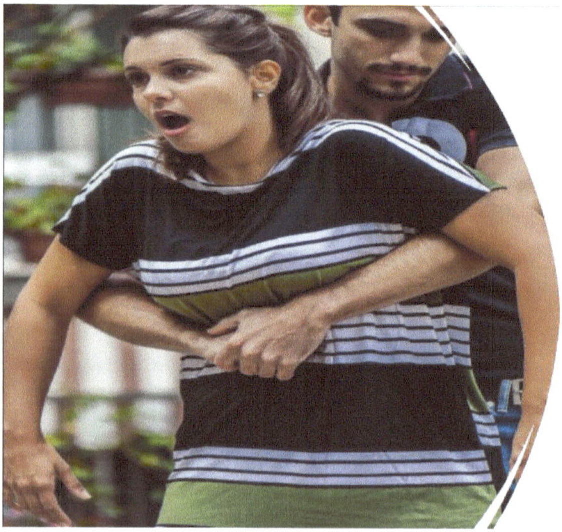

DENTAL PRACTICE CHOKING GUIDE

COMMON CAUSES IN PATIENTS

- Eating too quickly
- Loose or poorly fitting dentures
- Eating while lying down
- Not chewing properly
- Small objects, toys, or teeth
- Vomit

DENTAL INSTRUMENTS AND MATERIALS THAT CAN CAUSE CHOKING

- Root canal files
- Dental burs
- Cotton wool
- Water or saliva

- **Signs of a child choking**
-
- Suspect a foreign-body airway obstruction if a child or adolescent cannot speak, breathe, or cough effectively.
- **Call 999 or 112**
- Call **for help** if the obstruction persists or the patient shows signs of severe choking.

EMERGENCY ACTIONS FOR INFANTS (<1 YEAR)

How to help a choking child

Follow these steps if the child is choking:

1. CALL 999 FOR AN AMBULANCE

Ask for an ambulance and tell them the child is choking

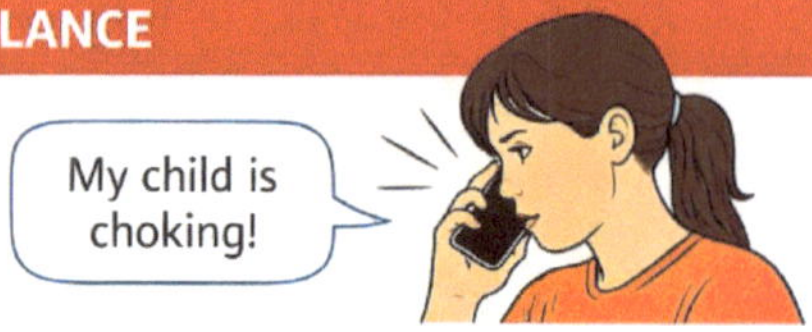

THEN

1. Give up to 5 back blows

Lean the child forward

Give 5 sharp back blows between the shoulder blades

Check if the choking is relieved after each blow

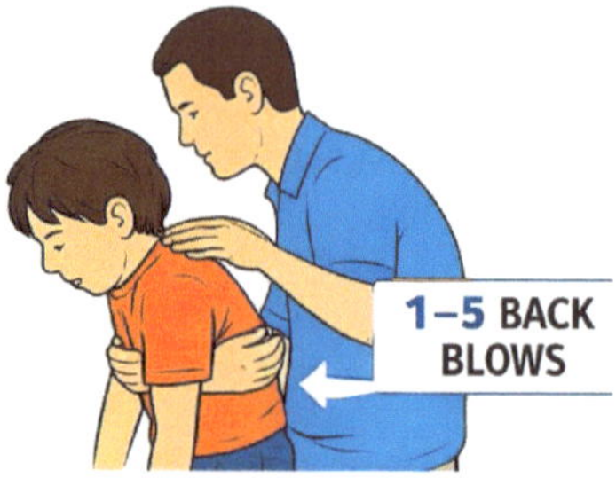

2. Give up to 5 back blows:

If still choking, give abdominal thrusts:

Stand behind the child

Place your fist in the middle of the abdomen

Pull inwards and upwards up to 5 times

Check if the choking is relieved after each thrust

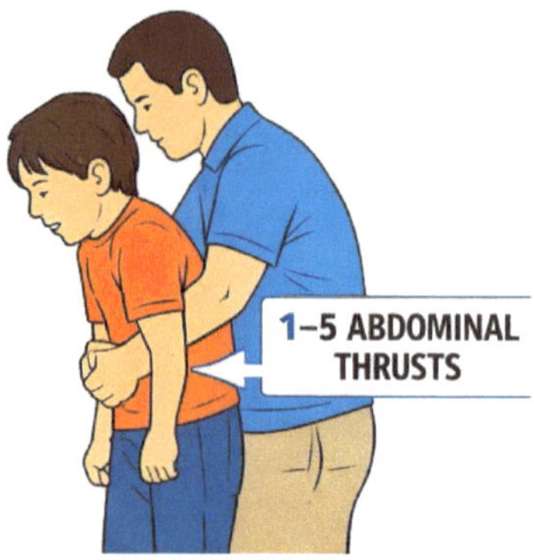

- ✓ Continue with 5 back blows and 5 abdominal thrusts
- ✓ Follow the call handler's advice until help arrives

KEY POINTS FOR DENTAL TEAMS

- Always **stop treatment immediately** if a patient starts choking.
- Keep the **airway clear of instruments, water, and saliva**.
- Ensure **oxygen and suction** are available in every clinical area.
- **AED should be immediately accessible**, including paediatric pads for children.
- Practice **regular training drills** for both adults and children.

SIGNS OF A CHOKING INFANT

- Suspect choking due to a foreign object when an infant cries aloud (infants or more minor children) when feeding, eating, or playing unsupervised.

CALL FOR 999 OR 112

- Call or have someone call the ambulance service as soon as possible.

GIVE 5 BACK BLOWS

Position the infant face down along your forearm, resting your arm on your thigh. Support the head and keep it lower than the chest. Deliver up to five sharp back blows between the shoulder blades, checking after each blow to see if the obstruction has cleared.

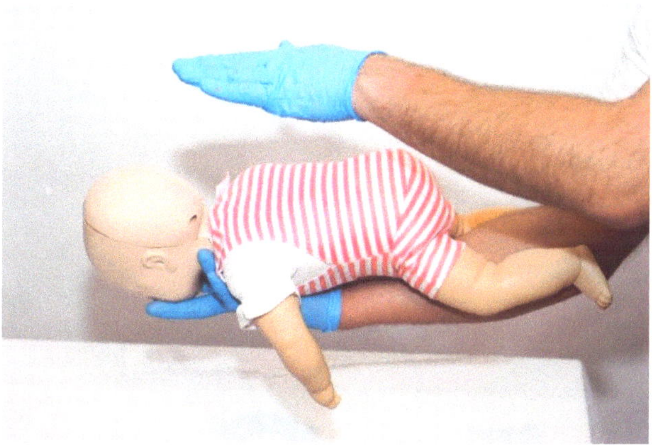

Chest Thrust with two thumbs encircling technique

Place the baby on their back on your lap. Wrap your hands around their chest and use your thumbs to give up to five quick pushes on the middle of the chest. Check after each push to see if the object has come out.

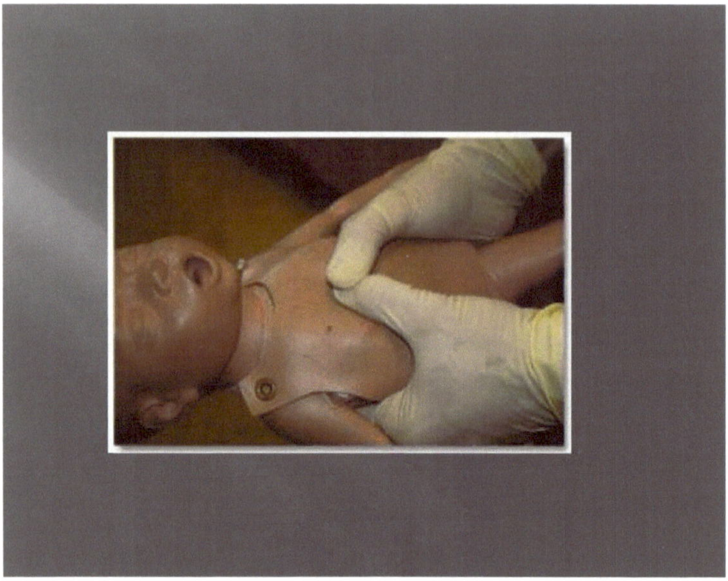

NO BLIND FINGER SWEEPS

Do not put your fingers blindly into the baby's mouth. Remove the object only if you can see it clearly.

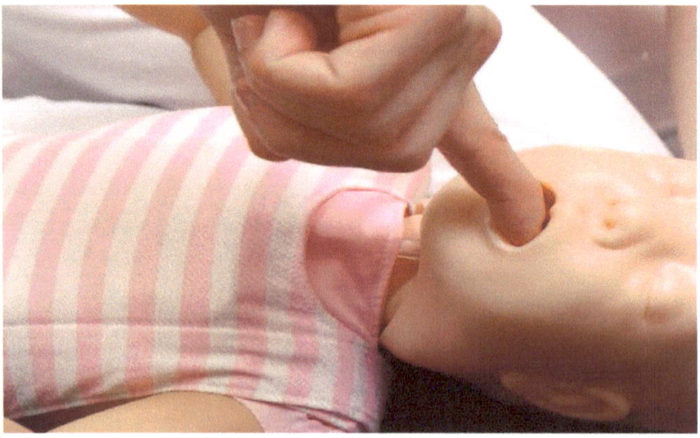

Do not put your fingers blindly into the baby's mouth. Remove the object only if you can see it clearly.

RESUSCITATION COUNCIL GUIDELINES ON THE USE OF SUCTION-BASED AIRWAY CLEARANCE DEVICES, SUCH AS LIFEVAC, FOR INDIVIDUALS CHOKING IN A DENTAL PRACTICE.

The Resuscitation Council does not yet support the use of these devices because:

a. There are insufficient evidence and research on the safety of these anti-choking devices.

b. There is no evidence that they are effective.

c. The use of the devices may delay the use of established treatments for choking.

d. Trained healthcare professionals already use advanced techniques such as suction, laryngoscopes, and forceps to remove foreign bodies stuck in the airway.

AUDITING RESUSCITATION EQUIPMENT (Dental & Clinical Settings)

- **Weekly equipment checks**
- Document findings
- Replace expired or faulty items
- Conduct **debriefs after any cardiac arrest**
- Take immediate corrective action

OXYGEN

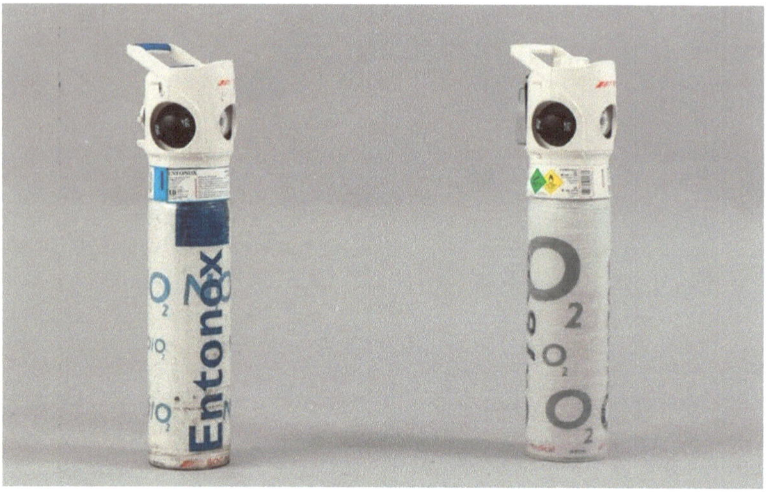

There are two main types of oxygen in clinical environments: oxygen and Entonox. The gases are compressed into cylinders of varied sizes.

Oxygen Equipment assembly

The components of an oxygen equipment bag are:

You will need a therapy mask, a resuscitation mask, tubing, a bag valve mask with a reservoir bag, a regulator, and a medical-grade oxygen cylinder. Lie the cylinder on the floor.

- Attach the tube from the non-rebreathe bag or bag valve mask to the oxygen tank
- The cylinder should be turned on

The flow rate should be set to 15 L/Min when treating a critical illness. Put a non-rebreather bag or a BVM mask over the patient's mouth and nose, and monitor them.

Disassembly of the oxygen cylinder.

- Remove the mask from the patient's face and ensure the gauge is off until the pressure is zero.

- The cylinder should be replaced with a new one

Oxygen delivery devices

Non-rebreathe bag: This delivers high-concentration oxygen (15 L). The device comprises a mask and a reservoir bag fitted with a one-way valve. The valve ensures oxygen is inhaled and exhaled air is not returned to the bag.

Simple face mask has ports on either side of the mask, which allow air to be sucked into the face mask.

OXYGEN CLASSIFICATION

Classification -Oxygen is a gas.

Action- helps the release of cellular energy.

Indications- hypoxia, ischaemic chest pain, respiratory illnesses, carbon monoxide poisoning, shock, and traumatic injuries

Adverse effects-

- High doses can lead to reduced levels of consciousness.
- High doses of oxygen to a COPD patient can lead to respiratory depression or patients with chronic carbon dioxide retention.
- Unnecessary high-concentration oxygen in normoxic patients may cause coronary vasoconstriction. Oxygen remains indicated for hypoxia and critical illness.

Contraindications- avoid giving oxygen to patients who have known paraquat poisoning. **Dosage**

Low-concentration oxygen

1-4 l/min by nasal cannula

High concentration

10-15 l/min administered through a non-rebreather mask.

Venturi Mask The Venturi mask has differently coloured spigots, allowing more accurate and adequate oxygen delivery at different concentrations. It is more effective for patients with COPD.

Nasal Cannula delivers oxygen through two nasal prongs

Nebuliser– used to deliver aerosolised drugs.

ASTHMA

Asthma is a chronic lung condition where the airways become inflamed and narrowed, causing breathing difficulties such as wheezing, coughing, and shortness of breath.

Asthma management can involve inhaled bronchodilators; when those prove ineffective, try intravenous (IV) medications. Both medications aim to reduce bronchospasm and lung inflammation.

A **reliever inhaler** is used to **quickly relieve asthma symptoms such as** wheezing, breathlessness, and chest tightness.
It works by **opening the airways** and provides relief within minutes.

Common examples include **salbutamol (blue inhaler)**.
It is used **when symptoms occur**, not every day.

RELIEVER INHALER

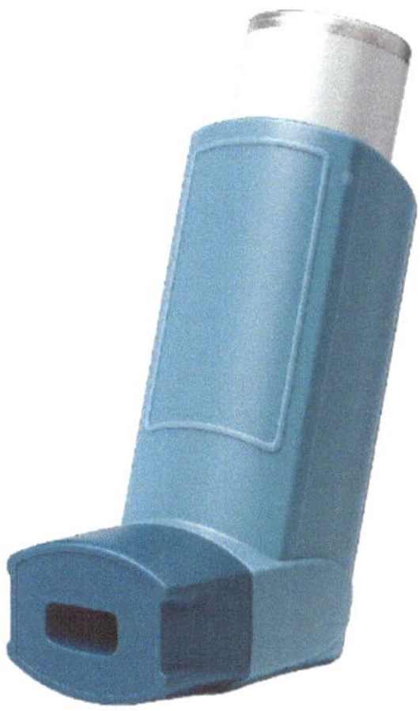

PREVENTER INHALER

A **preventer inhaler** is an asthma inhaler containing **inhaled corticosteroids** that is used **daily** to reduce airway inflammation and prevent asthma symptoms and attacks.

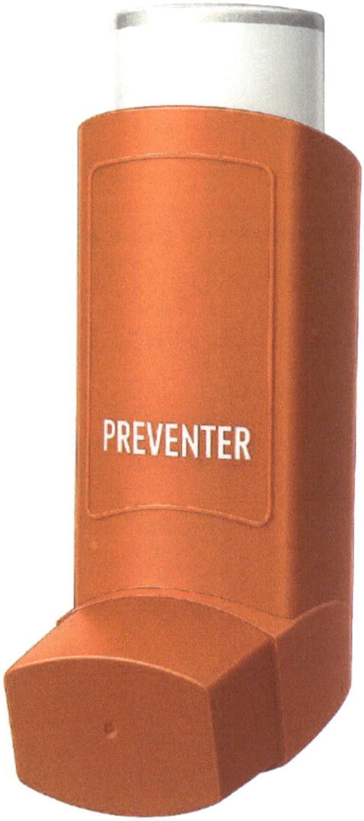

Salbutamol (β_2-Agonist Bronchodilator)

Overview

Salbutamol is a **short-acting β_2-adrenoceptor agonist (SABA)** used as **first-line treatment for acute bronchospasm**. It relaxes **smooth muscle in the lower airways**, leading to bronchodilation and improved airflow.

When delivered via **metered-dose inhaler (MDI) with a spacer or oxygen-driven nebuliser, salbutamol rapidly relieves bronchospasm and reduces the** work of breathing.

- **Onset:** 2–5 minutes
- **Peak effect:** 15–30 minutes
- **Duration:** 4–6 hours

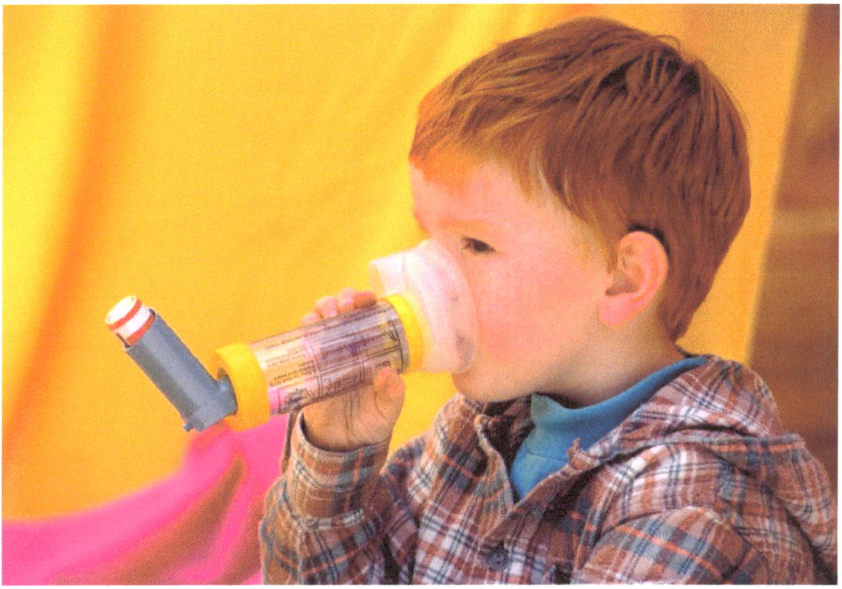

(Oxygen-driven nebulisers are recommended in **acute severe or life-threatening asthma** to avoid hypoxia.)

Presentations

- **MDI:** 100 micrograms per actuation
- **Nebuliser solution:** 2.5 mg / 5 mg (commonly 2.5 mg in 2.5 mL or 5 mg in 2.5 mL)

Indications

Salbutamol is indicated for:

- **Acute asthma exacerbation** (including severe and life-threatening asthma)
- **Acute bronchospasm** associated with:
    - Anaphylaxis
    - Allergic reactions
    - Smoke inhalation
    - COPD exacerbation with wheeze
- **Expiratory wheeze and respiratory distress**

Contraindications

- **No absolute contraindications in life-threatening emergencies**

Use with caution in:

- Known hypersensitivity to salbutamol
- Significant tachyarrhythmias
- Severe cardiovascular disease

Cautions

Use with caution in patients with:

- Ischaemic heart disease or arrhythmias
- Hypertension
- Hyperthyroidism
- Pregnancy (especially late pregnancy – may cause uterine relaxation)

- Concurrent **non-selective beta-blockers** (may reduce bronchodilator effect)

Common Side Effects

- Tremor
- Tachycardia
- Palpitations
- Headache
- Anxiety or agitation
- Muscle cramps
- Peripheral vasodilation
- Hypokalaemia (with high or repeated doses)

SALBUTAMOL – DOSING AND ADMINISTRATION

A. Salbutamol MDI (100 micrograms) with Spacer

Preferred first-line route where possible

Patient Group	Dose	Route	Repeat
Children <5 yrs	2–10 puffs	MDI + spacer	Every 10–20 minutes as needed
Children ≥5 yrs	2–10 puffs	MDI + spacer	Every 10–20 minutes as needed
Adults	2–10 puffs	MDI + spacer	Every 10–20 minutes as needed

Equivalence:
10 puffs ≈ 5 mg nebulised salbutamol

B. Salbutamol Nebuliser (Oxygen-Driven)

Used for **acute severe or life-threatening asthma**, or if MDI is ineffective or not tolerated.

Age Group	Dose	Route	Repeat
Children <5 yrs	2.5 mg	Oxygen-driven nebuliser	Every 20 minutes initially
Children 5–11 yrs	2.5–5 mg	Oxygen-driven nebuliser	Every 20 minutes initially
Children ≥12 yrs	5 mg	Oxygen-driven nebuliser	Every 15–30 minutes
Adults	5 mg	Oxygen-driven nebuliser	Every 15–30 minutes

Continuous nebulisation may be required in severe cases under medical supervision.

TERBUTALINE (Alternative β_2-Agonist)

(Used if salbutamol is unavailable or ineffective)

Age Group	Dose	Route	Repeat
<5 yrs	2.5 mg	Oxygen-driven nebuliser	Every 20–30 minutes
5–11 yrs	2.5–5 mg	Oxygen-driven nebuliser	Every 20–30 minutes
≥12 yrs	5 mg	Oxygen-driven nebuliser	Every 20–30 minutes
Adults	5 mg	Oxygen-driven nebuliser	Every 20–30 minutes

SYSTEMIC CORTICOSTEROIDS

Should be given **early in moderate-to-severe asthma exacerbations**.

PREDNISOLONE (Oral)

Patient Group	Dose	Route	Duration
Children <5 yrs	10 mg	Oral	3 days
Children 5–11 yrs	20 mg	Oral	3 days
Children 12–17 yrs	40–50 mg	Oral	At least 5 days
Adults	40–50 mg	Oral	At least 5 days

HYDROCORTISONE (IV – Sodium Succinate)

Used if the patient **cannot tolerate oral medication** or in **life-threatening asthma**.

Patient Group	Dose	Route	Frequency
<1 year	25 mg	IV	Every 6 hours
1–4 years	50 mg	IV	Every 6 hours
5–17 years	100 mg	IV	Every 6 hours
Adults	100 mg	IV	Every 6 hours

Switch to **oral prednisolone as soon as possible**.

IPRATROPIUM BROMIDE (Atrovent)

Add-on therapy for acute severe or life-threatening asthma

Patient Group	Dose	Route	Frequency
Children <12 yrs	250 micrograms	Oxygen-driven nebuliser	Every 20–30 min for 2 hrs, then 4–6 hourly
Children ≥12 yrs	500 micrograms	Oxygen-driven nebuliser	Every 4–6 hours
Adults	500 micrograms	Oxygen-driven nebuliser	Every 4–6 hours

Key Learning Points

- Use **MDI + spacer first** whenever possible
- Use **oxygen-driven nebulisers** in hypoxic patients
- **Early steroids save lives**
- Combine **salbutamol + ipratropium** in severe attacks
- Escalate early if **poor response after repeated bronchodilators**

ANAPHYLAXIS

Anaphylaxis is a **severe, rapid-onset, life-threatening allergic reaction** caused by the sudden release of mediators (like histamine) from mast cells and basophils. It can affect **multiple body systems** at once—especially the **airway, breathing, and circulation**—and requires **immediate emergency treatment**.

What happens in anaphylaxis

Anaphylaxis typically develops **within minutes** of exposure to an allergen and may include:

- **Airway:** throat tightness, swelling of tongue/lips, hoarseness, stridor
- **Breathing:** wheeze, shortness of breath, chest tightness
- **Circulation:** hypotension, dizziness, collapse, shock
- **Skin:** urticaria (hives), flushing, itching, angioedema
- **GI:** nausea, vomiting, abdominal cramps

Key point: Skin signs may be absent—do not rule out anaphylaxis if airway or circulatory symptoms are present.

Common causes of anaphylaxis in a dental practice

1. Local anaesthetics (rare, but important)

- True allergy is **rare**
- Reactions are more commonly due to:
    - **Preservatives** (e.g., sulphites)
    - **Latex contamination** of cartridges
- Ester-type LAs (rarely used) have a higher allergy risk than amide types

2. Antibiotics

- **Penicillin and cephalosporins** (most common)

- Can occur even if the patient has taken them before without problems

3. Latex

- Gloves, rubber dams, elastic bands
- Higher risk in:
  - Patients with multiple surgeries
  - Spina bifida
  - Healthcare workers
- Symptoms may worsen with repeated exposure during treatment

4. Chlorhexidine

- Found in:
  - Mouthwashes
  - Gels
  - Impregnated dressings
- Increasingly recognized cause of **peri-procedural anaphylaxis**

5. Analgesics

- **NSAIDs** (e.g., ibuprofen, aspirin)
- Can trigger anaphylaxis or severe bronchospasm in susceptible patients

6. Other potential triggers

- Acrylics, impression materials (rare)
- Flavouring agents or additives
- Topical antibiotics

Why this matters in dentistry

- Anaphylaxis is **unpredictable**
- Can occur **even without a known allergy**

- Dental teams must be prepared for **immediate recognition and management**, including:
    - Prompt use of **IM adrenaline (epinephrine)**
    - Calling emergency services
    - Airway and oxygen support

Dental Anaphylaxis Recognition Checklist

Suspect ANAPHYLAXIS if there is:

Sudden onset (minutes) after exposure *PLUS* **airway, breathing or circulation compromise**

Airway (A)

☐ Throat tightness

☐ Hoarse voice / difficulty speaking

☐ Swollen tongue, lips, or face

☐ Stridor

Breathing (B)

☐ Shortness of breath

☐ Wheeze / bronchospasm

☐ Rapid breathing

☐ Cyanosis

☐ SpO_2 falling

Circulation (C)

☐ Dizziness or collapse

☐ Hypotension

☐ Tachycardia

☐ Pale, clammy skin

☐ Loss of consciousness

Skin / Mucosa (may be absent)

☐ Urticaria (hives)

☐ Flushing

☐ Itching

☐ Angioedema

Dental Anaphylaxis Emergency Protocol

IMMEDIATE ACTIONS (ABCDE approach)

1. STOP treatment

- Remove allergen
- Lie the patient **flat** unless they are struggling to breathe while lying on their back
- If breathing difficulty, get them to sit in a **semi-reclined position**
- If pregnant, put the patient in a **left lateral tilt**

2. CALL FOR HELP

- Shout for assistance
- **Call 999or 112 immediately**

3. ADRENALINE (Epinephrine) – FIRST LINE OF TREATMENT

Do NOT delay

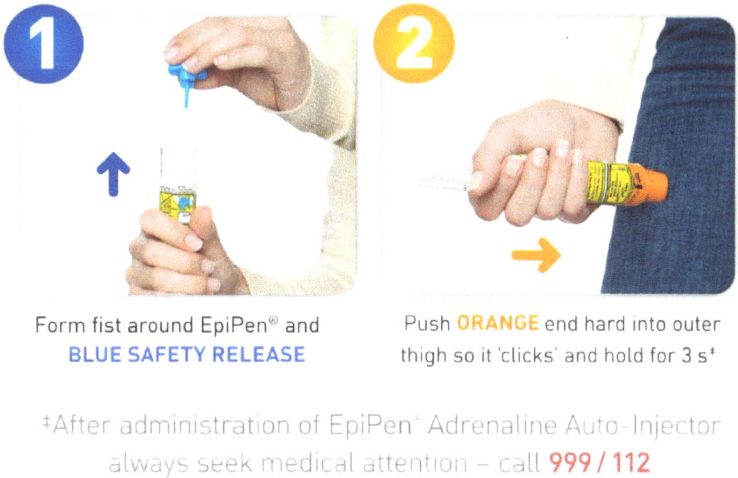
1
2
Form fist around EpiPen® and
BLUE SAFETY RELEASE
Push ORANGE end hard into outer
thigh so it 'clicks' and hold for 3 s‡
‡After administration of EpiPen® Adrenaline Auto-Injector
always seek medical attention – call 999 / 112

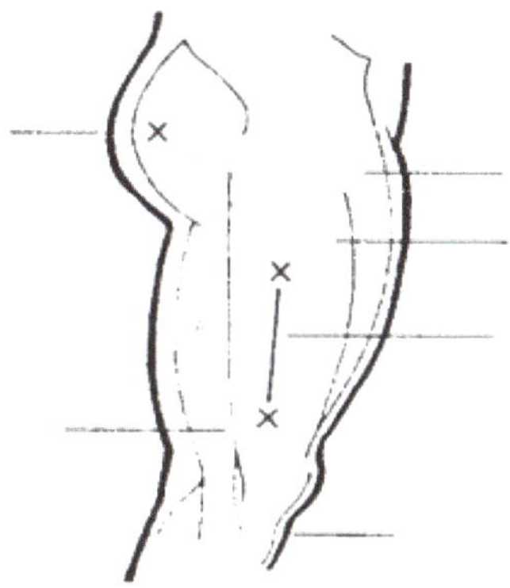

Route:

Intramuscular (IM)
Anterolateral thigh (vastus lateralis)

HOW TO USE THE EPIPEN

STEP 1

Form your fist around the EpiPen and remove the safety cap by pulling it straight up.

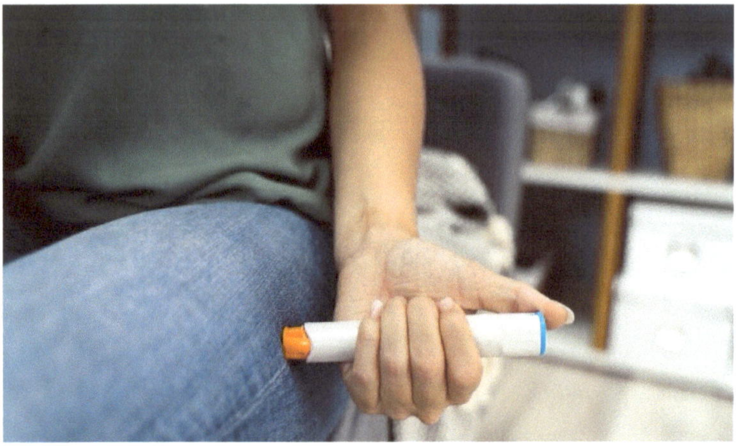

STEP 2

Swing and push the orange part of the auto-injector firmly against the anterolateral thigh until it "clicks." Hold the injection in place for 3 seconds. Count "1,2,3" slowly.

STEP 3

After injection, the orange cover automatically extends to ensure the needle is never exposed.

STEP 4

Isolate the casualty from the trigger.

Make sure the casualty is isolated from the trigger. Remove the stinger stuck to the skin if a bee has stung the casualty.

RECOMMENDED NEEDLE LENGTH

The resuscitation council recommends that the length be 25mm for all ages, based on a recommendation from Public Health England.[1]

Dental practice should have adrenaline 1:1000 (1mg/ml) ampoules in their emergency drugs kit. Anaphylaxis packs should have the following:

---

[1] Public Health England. Immunisation against infectious disease. 2014. Available online at https://www.gov.uk/government/collections/immunisation-against-infectious-disease-the-green-book (accessed April 2020).

- Adrenaline 1:1000 ampoules x 2
- Blue 23G 25 mm needles x 4
- Graduated 1 ml syringes x 4.

Some dental practices prefer pre-filled syringes. The advantage of the pre-filled syringes is that they prevent the need to draw the medication from an ampoule.

The injection should be administered in the anterolateral aspect of the middle third of the thigh, but if that is not possible, it should be administered on the arm.

ADRENALINE AUTO INJECTOR OR AMPOULES-WHICH IS BETTER FOR TREATING ANAPHYLAXIS?

It is up to the individual clinical environment to determine whether to use the ampoule or an adrenaline auto-injector. The ampoules are cheaper, and their supply is more dependable as they are not prone to the supply chain issues that affect adrenaline auto-injectors. The needles are longer, and it is necessary to give the appropriate dose, especially for obese patients. In the heat of the moment, drawing the right amounts of adrenaline from an ampoule with a syringe may be problematic. Errors are sometimes unavoidable.

Adrenaline auto-injectors are made for self-use by patients and are prescribed for each patient. They are expensive and have a limited shelf life. Most auto-injectors deliver 300 mcg of adrenaline to adults, less than the recommended dose for adults and teenagers, which is 500 mcg.

The needles for the standard auto-injectors are not long enough for some patients. For example, the EpiPen has a 16 mm needle to administer 300 mcg. The Resuscitation Council recommends that a standard blue needle (25mm and 23G) be used to inject intramuscular adrenaline. Still, a longer needle (38 mm in length and 21 G) may be needed for larger patients.

GRADUATED ADRENALINE, SYRINGE, AND NEEDLE

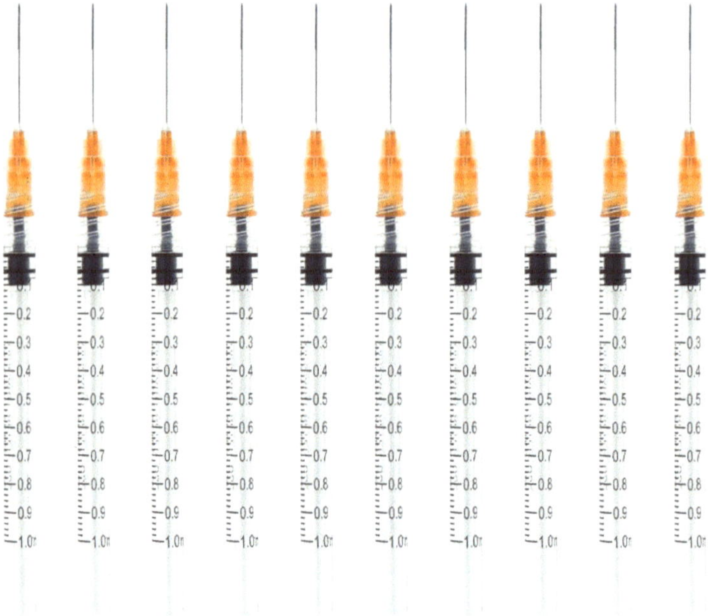

THE AMPOULE-1: 1000

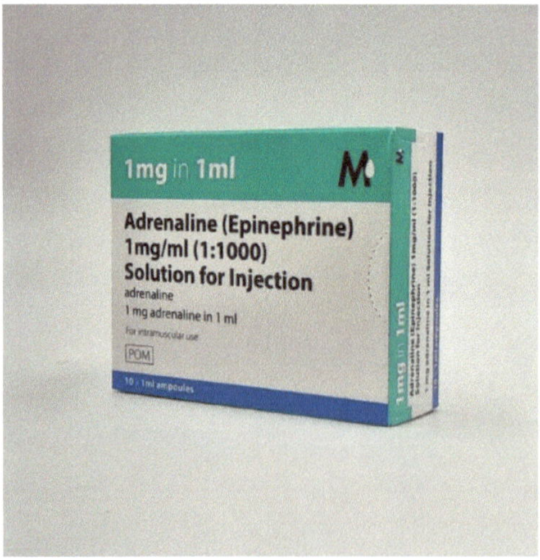

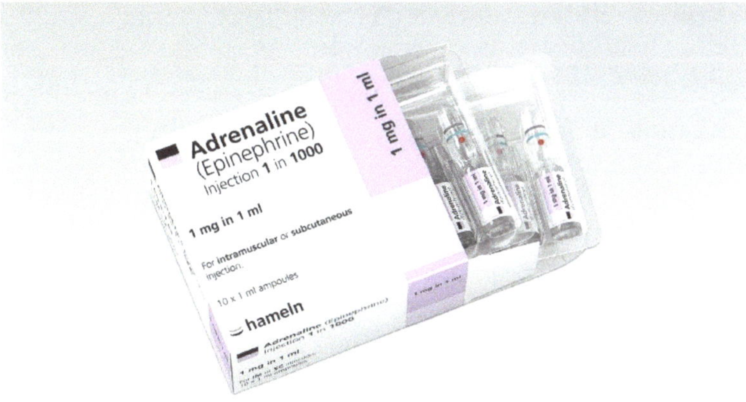

Adrenaline Dosing (IM)

Patient	Dose	Concentration
Adult	500 mcg	1:1000 (1 mg/mL)
Child 6–12 yrs	300 mcg	1:1000 (1 mg/mL)
Child >6mths-<6yrs	150 mcg	1:1000(1mg/mL)
Infant 0-6mths	100 mcg	1: 1000 (mg/mL)

Repeat every 5 minutes if no improvement.

4. AIRWAY & BREATHING SUPPORT

☐ High-flow **oxygen (15 L/min)** via mask

☐ Prepare suction

☐ Monitor SpO_2

☐ Be ready for airway obstruction

5. CIRCULATION

☐ Keep patient warm

☐ Monitor pulse & BP

☐ If trained and available → IV fluids

SECONDARY MEDICATIONS (Do NOT delay adrenaline)

(Given after adrenaline)

- **Antihistamine** (e.g. chlorphenamine or cetirizine)

  Antihistamines do not treat airway, breathing, or circulatory compromise and must not delay adrenaline. They may be used later for cutaneous symptoms once the patient is stable.

- **Corticosteroid** (e.g. hydrocortisone)- routine administration of corticosteroid is not advised because there is no reliable evidence that they improve outcomes or prevent biphasic reactions.

- **Salbutamol** for persistent bronchospasm. It must not be used instead of adrenaline, but can be administered where there is persistent bronchospasm despite administering adrenaline

OBSERVATION & HANDOVER

- Patient **must be transferred to hospital**
- Risk of **biphasic reaction** (up to 24 hrs)
- Document:
  - Trigger
  - Time of onset
  - Drugs & doses
  - Response

Common Pitfalls in Dental Settings

✗ Delaying adrenaline

✗ Confusing anaphylaxis with vasovagal syncope

✗ Sitting patient upright with hypotension. Please encourage them to lie down and raise their legs. But if they struggle to breathe lying on their backs, have them sit in a comfortable position.

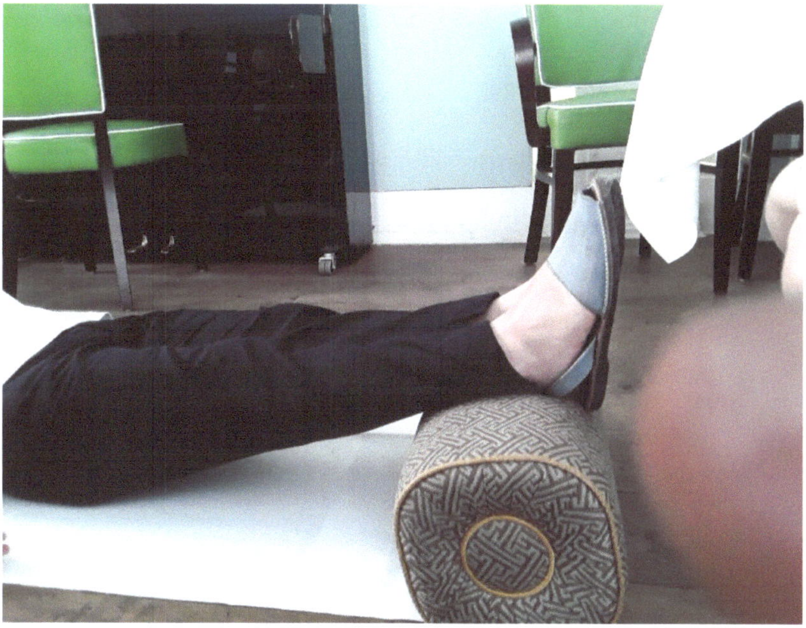

WHO CAN ADMINISTER THE ADENALINE AMPOULES?

Legal Basis for Emergency Adrenaline Use

Under the **Prescription Only Medicines (Human Use) Order 1997**, certain injectable drugs (including **adrenaline for anaphylaxis**) *may be administered by anyone in a **life-saving emergency*** to save a life, even **without a prescription**. This includes adrenaline ampoules drawn up and given by syringe and needle.[2]

Who Can Administer Adrenaline Ampoules in a Dental Practice

1. Dentists

✓ **Always permitted** to administer adrenaline ampoules intramuscularly in a medical emergency

✓ Must be trained and competent in drawing up and administering IM injections

---

[2] psm.sdcep.org.uk

As registered clinicians, dentists have clinical autonomy and are responsible for providing emergency care, including intramuscular adrenaline for **anaphylaxis**.[3]

2. Dental Hygienists and Dental Therapists

✓ **Can administer adrenaline** IF:

- They are **competent and trained** in emergency management and IM injections
- They are working **within their scope of practice** and local protocols

The **GDC** references Resuscitation Council guidance, which forms the standard for emergency drugs and training. Hygienists/therapists may hold and use emergency drugs on site, but must have appropriate training and protocols in place. (General Dental Council)

Note: Direct drug supply/administration rules are evolving, but in emergencies, the *Prescription Only Medicines (Human Use) Order* allows life-saving use irrespective of prescription status. (psm.sdcep.org.uk)

3. Dental Nurses and Other Team Members

✓ **May administer adrenaline ampoules** *in a life-saving emergency* if:

- They are **trained and competent** in emergency procedures
- They act under the **practice's medical emergency protocol and supervision**
- The situation is **a genuine anaphylactic emergency**

Resuscitation Council UK and SDCEP both make it clear that *anyone present who is competent* can administer adrenaline in anaphylaxis to save a life. (psm.sdcep.org.uk)

Important Clarifications

Training & Competence

[3] General Dental Council

All team members who **might administer adrenaline ampoules** must be:

- **Trained** in medical emergencies, including anaphylaxis recognition and IM injection
- **Practised regularly** with mock scenarios
- Up-to-date with resuscitation skills as expected by the Resuscitation Council and GDC standards (General Dental Council)

The GDC states that *every registrant must know their role in a medical emergency and be sufficiently trained and competent to perform it.* (cpd4dentalnurses.co.uk)

*The Prescription Only Medicines (Human Use) Order 1997 [1] lists injectable drugs that can be administered by anyone for the purpose of saving a life in an emergency; this includes adrenaline and glucagon. Therefore, all dental team members may administer adrenaline and glucagon, and the non-injectable drugs listed below. However, dental team members must be competent in the use of these drugs, and employers must accept responsibility for the actions of staff." (SDCEP-The Scottish Dental SDCEP Clinical effectiveness Programme)

- Examples of the injectable drugs listed are Adrenaline, 1 ml ampoules or pre-filled syringes of 1:1000 solution for intramuscular injection.
- Glucagon, for intramuscular injection of 1 mg.

"Dental practices might wish to stock the following to aid the management of patients with mild allergic reactions

- Cetirizine, 10 mg tablets, or oral solution (5 mg/5 ml).
- Chlorphenamine, 4 mg tablets or oral solution (2 mg/5 ml); (NB: chlorphenamine can cause drowsiness)

Loratadine, 10 mg tablets or syrup (5 mg/5 ml)." (SDCEP-The Scottish Dental Clinical Effectiveness Programme)

Human Medicines Regulations 2012

Use of Intramuscular Adrenaline by Anyone

◆ The Key Legal Provision

The relevant part of the Human Medicines Regulations 2012 is **Regulation 238**
(*Exemptions for the administration of prescription-only medicines in an emergency*).

What the Law Explicitly Allows

Regulation 238 permits:

Any person to administer a **Prescription Only Medicine (POM)**
by injection
for the purpose of saving life
in an emergency

This exemption applies **even if**:

- The person is **not a prescriber**
- The medicine is normally **prescription-only**
- There is **no Patient Specific Direction (PSD)** or **Patient Group Direction (PGD)**

How This Applies to Adrenaline

- **Adrenaline (epinephrine)** is a **Prescription Only Medicine**
- IM adrenaline is the **first-line treatment for anaphylaxis**
- Anaphylaxis is a **life-threatening emergency**

→ Therefore, **any person** may legally administer **IM adrenaline** in an emergency **to save life**, provided the situation is genuine.

Application in a Dental Practice

Under **HMR 2012 Regulation 238**:

The following may administer IM adrenaline in anaphylaxis:

- Dentists
- Dental hygienists
- Dental therapists

- Dental nurses
- Any other trained person present

✓ **No prescription required**

✓ **No PGD required**

✓ **No professional registration required**

The legal authority comes **directly from the Regulations**, not from professional scope alone.

Important Conditions and Safeguards

Although legally permitted, the following still apply:

1️⃣ **Emergency Only**

- Must be a **life-threatening situation**
- Routine or precautionary use is **not covered**

2️⃣ **Route Matters**

- IM adrenaline is appropriate
- **IV adrenaline is NOT covered** and is unsafe in primary care

3️⃣ **Professional Accountability**

- GDC standards still apply:
    - Act within competence
    - Be trained
    - Be able to justify actions

The exemption allows administration, **not poor practice**.

Alignment with National Guidance

Resuscitation Council (UK)

- Explicitly supports **IM adrenaline by trained responders**
- Emphasises **do not delay adrenaline**

NICE / BNF

- Recognises adrenaline as **first-line** for anaphylaxis

- Notes emergency use without prescription

GDC

- Requires registrants to:
    - Know their role in emergencies
    - Be trained and competent
    - Act in patients' best interests

HMR 2012 provides the **legal permission**; professional bodies provide the **practice standards**.

Summary Table

Team Member	Can administer adrenaline ampoule?	Conditions
Dentist	Yes	Always, with training
Hygienist / Therapist	Yes	With training + within scope + protocols
Dental Nurse / Other	Yes	In a true emergency with competency & practice protocol
Clinical Dental Technician	Not expected to hold/administer emergency kit medicines	GDC does *not* expect CDTs to have emergency drug kits[4] (General Dental Council)

[4] General Dental Council

CQC / GDC Compliance Checklist – Medical Emergencies & Adrenaline Use

Practice Name: ____________________________ Date of Audit: ____________________________

Governance & Policies	
Written medical emergencies policy in place	■
Policy includes anaphylaxis & adrenaline ampoules	■
Policy reviewed annually	■
Emergency Drugs & Equipment	
Adrenaline 1:1000 ampoules available and in-date	■
Syringes & IM needles available	■
Oxygen with masks and tubing available	■
Emergency drugs checked regularly	■
Training & Competence	
All clinical staff trained annually	■
Training includes IM adrenaline administration	■
Emergency drills carried out	■
Documentation & Review	
Emergency incidents documented	■
Significant events reviewed and learning shared	■

Audit completed by: ____________________________ Signature: ____________________________

NASAL ADRENALINE SPRAY FOR ANAPHYLAXIS

What is EURneffy®?

EURneffy® is a **needle-free adrenaline (epinephrine) nasal spray** used for the **emergency treatment of severe allergic reactions (anaphylaxis)**. It offers an alternative to traditional adrenaline auto-injectors (AAIs). [5]

Why it matters:
Fast administration of adrenaline during anaphylaxis saves lives. A nasal spray may reduce hesitation to treat because it **avoids needles** and can be **used[6] quickly** in emergencies.

Regulatory Status

- GB **Approved by the UK's MHRA (July 2025)** — first needle-free option for anaphylaxis in the UK for adults and children ≥ 30 kg. Expected to be **available now (late 2025)**. (
- EU **Approved by the European Commission (2024)** — authorised across EU Member States.

Who Can Use It?

Adults and **children weighing 30 kg or more**
Prescription-only medicine — must be prescribed by a healthcare professional. [7]

How It Works (Quick Summary)

- A **single-use nasal spray** containing **2 mg adrenaline**.[8]
- Delivered **into one nostril only** — ready to use with no priming needed. (EURneffy®)

---

[5] GOV.UK

[7] Anaphylaxis Campaign
[8] EURneffy®

- Adrenaline is absorbed through the nasal lining and enters the bloodstream quickly to counteract anaphylaxis.[9]

When to Use It

Use EURneffy **as soon as signs of anaphylaxis appear**, such as:

- Difficulty breathing or wheeze
- Throat tightness or swelling
- Light-headedness/collapse
- Rapid onset of hives and low blood pressure

Administer immediately and call 999 — adrenaline is time-critical in anaphylaxis. [10]

Important Dosing & Administration Notes

✓ **One dose per device.** After use, the device must be discarded. [11]

✓ **Carry two devices** at all times — a second dose may be needed if symptoms continue or worsen.[12]

✓ **Seek urgent medical help after use**, even if symptoms improve[13]

Compared to Auto-Injectors

Advantages

- **Needle-free** — easier use for some patients
- **Smaller and lighter** to carry
- **Better temperature stability** and potentially longer shelf life than some auto-injectors [14]

---

9 Anaphylaxis Campaign
10 European Medicines Agency (EMA)
11 EURneffy®
12 (Anaphylaxis Campaign)

13(European Medicines Agency (EMA))

14 (Pharma Focus Europe)

Note: Traditional auto-injectors remain widely used and established; EURneffy is an additional option. Proper training in all adrenaline-delivery methods remains essential.

Safety & Side Effects

Common reported effects may include:

- Nasal discomfort or irritation
- Headache or congestion
- Throat irritation
- Nervousness, dizziness
  (*Common side effects seen with nasal adrenaline sprays in general — see full prescribing info for details.*) [15]

Key Learner Takeaways

- EURneffy is a **needle-free adrenaline spray** for emergency anaphylaxis treatment.
- Approved in the **UK and EU** for adults and children ≥ 30 kg.
- **Use immediately** on the first signs of anaphylaxis and **call emergency services**.
- Always **carry two devices**.
- Does **not replace emergency medical care** — hospital assessment is needed after use.

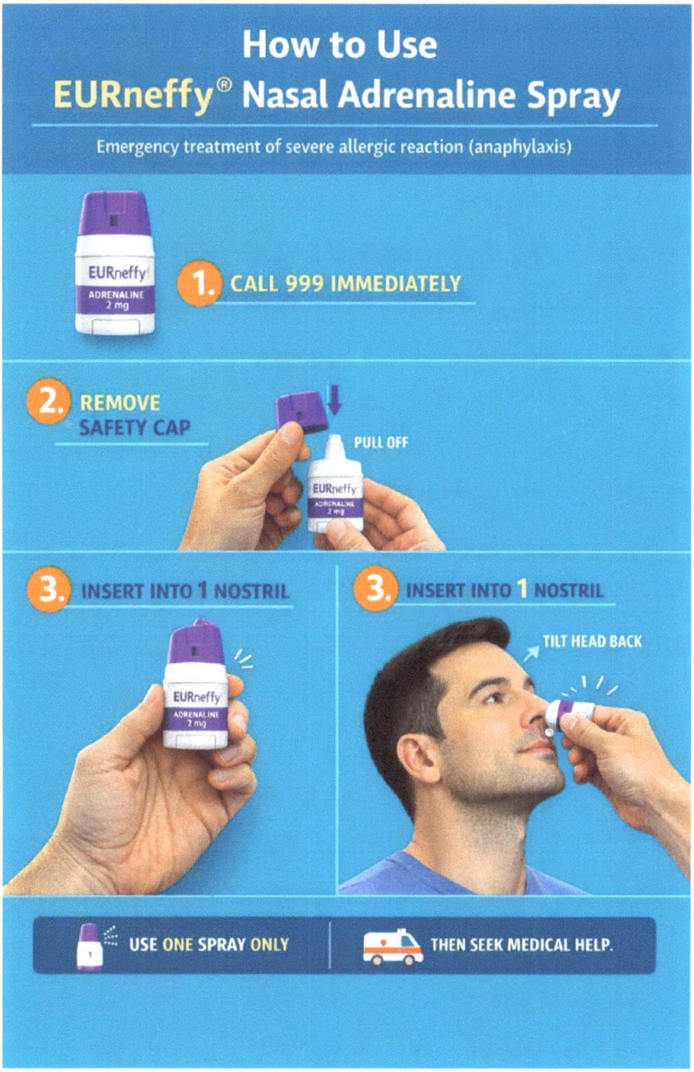
How to Use
EURneffy® Nasal Adrenaline Spray
Emergency treatment of severe allergic reaction (anaphylaxis)
1. CALL 999 IMMEDIATELY
2. REMOVE SAFETY CAP
PULL OFF
3. INSERT INTO 1 NOSTRIL
3. INSERT INTO 1 NOSTRIL
TILT HEAD BACK
USE ONE SPRAY ONLY
THEN SEEK MEDICAL HELP.

Use of Adrenaline Auto-Injectors Prescribed for a Named Patient

Is it permissible to administer an adrenaline auto-injector prescribed for one individual to a different patient?

No.

Under current UK medicines legislation, an **adrenaline auto-injector (AAI) that has been prescribed for a named individual may only be administered to that named person**.

Although **anyone may administer adrenaline to save a life in an emergency**, this legal exemption **does not extend to using a Prescription Only Medicine that has been specifically prescribed to someone else** when that medicine is an **adrenaline auto-injector**.

Legal Position (Summary)

- **Adrenaline (epinephrine)** is a Prescription Only Medicine (POM).
- **Human Medicines Regulations 2012 (Regulation 238)** allow *any person* to administer a POM **by injection** in a life-threatening emergency **to save life**.
- However, this exemption **does not permit the use of a patient-specific prescribed medicine on another person** when that medicine is an **adrenaline auto-injector**.

Resuscitation Council (UK) Statement

"Currently, the law does not allow a non-prescriber to administer an adrenaline auto-injector which has been specifically prescribed for a named person to someone other than the person for whom it has been prescribed."

— **Resuscitation Council (UK)**

This position is consistently reflected in national dental and medical emergency guidance.

Practical Examples in a Dental Practice

Permitted

- Any trained person may administer:
    - **Practice-owned adrenaline auto-injector**, or
    - **Practice-owned adrenaline ampoule (1:1000) IM**
- A patient's **own prescribed auto-injector** may be used **on that same patient**.

Not Permitted

- Using **Patient B's prescribed adrenaline auto-injector** to treat **Patient A**, even in an emergency.

Example Scenario

- Patient A develops anaphylaxis during dental treatment.
- Patient B (in the waiting room) has a prescribed adrenaline auto-injector.

Unlawful: Using Patient B's auto-injector on Patient A
Lawful:

- Using the **practice's emergency adrenaline auto-injector**, or
- Drawing up and administering **IM adrenaline from a practice-held ampoule**

Key Compliance Message for Practices

Dental practices must:

- Stock **practice-owned adrenaline auto-injectors and/or adrenaline ampoules**
- Ensure staff are trained to:
    - Recognise anaphylaxis
    - Administer IM adrenaline promptly
- Avoid reliance on **patient-specific prescribed medicines for other patients**

HYPERVENTILATION (Acute over-breathing / anxiety-related breathlessness)

What it is

Hyperventilation is **breathing faster and/or deeper than the body's metabolic needs** (often triggered by **panic, anxiety, pain, or fear**). This can lead to **excessive "blowing off" of carbon dioxide, which may cause light-headedness, tingling, and carpopedal spasm (cramping in the hands/feet**).

In respiratory guidance, this often sits within **disordered breathing/hyperventilation syndrome**, where symptoms can **mimic asthma** and other cardiopulmonary problems—so assessment matters.[16]

Signs and symptoms (common)

- Feeling unable to "get a deep breath"
- **Dizziness/light-headedness**
- **Tingling or numbness** (around mouth, fingers)
- **Palpitations**
- Chest tightness or chest pain (often non-cardiac, but treat cautiously)
- **Dry mouth**
- Trembling, sweating
- **Carpopedal spasm** (spasms/cramps in hands/feet)
- Anxiety, fear, tearfulness

Management in a dental practice

1) First: assess for serious causes (do not assume anxiety)

Use an **ABCDE approach** and check **vital signs** (respiratory rate, pulse, BP, temperature, level of consciousness, oxygen saturation if available). The

---

[16] British Thoracic Society

NICE CKS on breathlessness emphasises an initial ABC assessment and deciding whether emergency admission is needed[17].

Red flags → call 999/112 (treat as an emergency until proven otherwise):

- Low SpO_2, cyanosis, severe wheeze/stridor
- Hypotension, collapse, altered consciousness
- Signs of anaphylaxis, severe asthma, chest pain suggestive of cardiac cause

2) Reassure and coach breathing (main treatment)

- Stop treatment, sit the patient **upright** and encourage relaxation.
- Use **calm reassurance** ("This is frightening but it will pass; I'll coach your breathing.")
- Coach **slow, controlled breathing**, for example:
    - **Pursed-lip breathing** (inhale gently through nose, exhale slowly through pursed lips)
    - Encourage slower rate and smaller breaths (avoid deep "gulping" breaths)

Breathing retraining that focuses on **reducing respiratory rate and/or tidal volume** is recommended as **first-line** for hyperventilation syndrome/disordered breathing.[18]

You can also use a simple cadence:
"In…2…3… Out…2…3…4…5" (longer out-breath)

3) Oxygen: only if indicated

If oxygen saturation is normal (94–98%), reassurance and breathing control are first-line. BTS guidance stresses oxygen should be used appropriately and targeted to need (i.e., treat hypoxaemia rather than anxiety symptoms)[19] (British Thoracic Society)

---

17 CKS

18 . (British Thoracic Society

19 British Thoracic Society

4) Avoid paper-bag rebreathing

Do **not** use paper-bag breathing in clinical settings: it risks worsening unrecognised **hypoxia** or other serious conditions presenting as "hyperventilation." (This is widely reflected in modern emergency care teaching; in dentistry, focus on assessment + coached breathing rather than rebreathing.)

SEIZURES: CLINICAL ASSESSMENT AND EMERGENCY MANAGEMENT

1. Definition of a Seizure

A seizure is a **sudden, excessive, and abnormal electrical discharge in the brain** that causes temporary changes in movement, behaviour, sensation, awareness, or consciousness.

Seizure type depends on:

- The **area of the brain involved**
- Whether the abnormal electrical activity remains focal or becomes generalised

2. Generalised Tonic–Clonic Seizures (GTCS)

Generalised tonic–clonic seizures are the most common type.

Clinical Features

- **Tonic phase**: sudden loss of consciousness with body stiffening
- **Clonic phase**: rhythmic jerking of limbs
- Eyes usually **open**, often rolled upwards
- Unresponsive to verbal commands or painful stimuli
- Tongue biting, drooling, cyanosis, and urinary incontinence

Duration

- Most seizures stop spontaneously within **60–90 seconds**
- Followed by a **post-ictal phase** of confusion, drowsiness, and fatigue

3. Epilepsy

Epilepsy is a **chronic neurological condition** characterised by a **predisposition to recurrent, unprovoked seizures**.

Common Causes or Triggers

- Stroke or traumatic brain injury
- Alcohol withdrawal or intoxication

- Hypoglycaemia
- Drug overdose or toxicity
- Central nervous system infection

4. Convulsive Status Epilepticus

Convulsive status epilepticus is defined as:

- A tonic–clonic seizure lasting **5 minutes or more**, **OR**
- Recurrent tonic–clonic seizures without full recovery of consciousness between episodes

This is a life-threatening medical emergency requiring immediate treatment.

5. Focal Seizures (With or Without Impaired Awareness)

- Originate in **one area of the brain**
- May remain focal or **progress to a generalised tonic–clonic seizure**
- Often preceded by an **aura**

Clinical Significance

- Treat as a tonic–clonic seizure if:
    - Consciousness is impaired **and**
    - The seizure lasts **5 minutes or more**
- Prolonged focal seizures (>60 minutes) increase the risk of permanent neurological injury

6. Phases of a Seizure

A. Prodromal Phase (Hours to Days Before)

Not experienced by all patients.

Common features

- Mood or behavioural changes
- Anxiety or irritability
- Sleep disturbance

- Fatigue or reduced concentration

B. Aura (Early Ictal Phase)

An aura is the **earliest manifestation of a focal seizure** and may act as a warning.

Symptoms

- Déjà vu or jamais vu
- Unusual smells, tastes, or sounds
- Visual disturbance
- Dizziness
- Numbness or pins and needles
- Nausea or headache
- Sudden fear or panic

C. Ictal Phase

The period of **active seizure activity**.

Signs

- Loss or alteration of consciousness
- Involuntary movements or twitching
- Abnormal speech or sounds
- Lip smacking or chewing
- Sudden loss of muscle tone or rigidity

D. Post-Ictal Phase (Recovery Phase)

Occurs after seizure activity ends.

Common features

- Confusion or disorientation
- Drowsiness or exhaustion
- Headache

- Nausea or thirst
- Temporary focal weakness (Todd's paresis)
- Urinary or bowel incontinence
- Emotional distress (fear, embarrassment, frustration)

7. Assessment and Initial Management

Safety and Positioning

- Ensure scene safety
- Protect the person from injury
- Once seizure activity stops, place the patient in the **recovery position** to maintain airway patency

History

- Witness account and estimated seizure duration
- Known epilepsy diagnosis
- Previous or recent seizures
- Preceding symptoms or triggers
- Alcohol or drug use
- Pregnancy status
- Past medical history and medications

Airway

- Maintain airway patency
- Use an **oropharyngeal airway** only if tolerated
- Use a **nasopharyngeal airway** unless facial trauma or basal skull fracture is suspected

Breathing

- Assess respiratory rate, effort, and oxygen saturation
- Administer **high-flow oxygen (15 L/min)** during tonic–clonic seizures

- Target oxygen saturation:
  - **94–98%** (most adults)
  - **88–92%** (COPD)
- Assist ventilation with **BVM and airway adjuncts** if required
- **Do not delay benzodiazepine administration** during ongoing convulsions

Circulation and Injuries

- Check pulse and capillary blood glucose
- Look for:
  - Head injury
  - Tongue biting
  - Urinary incontinence
  - Non-blanching rash (meningitis)
- In females of childbearing age, consider pregnancy and eclampsia

8. Emergency Drug Treatment: Prolonged Seizures

Indications for Benzodiazepines

Administer emergency benzodiazepines if:

- Seizure activity lasts **5 minutes or more**, OR
- **3 or more seizures occur within 1 hour**, OR
- There is ongoing seizure activity without recovery

9. Buccal Midazolam

Presentation

- Pre-filled oromucosal syringes:
  - **2.5 mg, 5 mg, 7.5 mg, or 10 mg**

Administration

- Buccal (between gum and cheek)

- May be repeated **once after 5–10 minutes** if seizures persist, in line with local protocol

10. Rectal Diazepam

Indication

- Prolonged convulsive seizures when buccal midazolam is unavailable or contraindicated

Diazepam Rectal Solution (2 mg/mL or 4 mg/mL)

Age group	Route	Dose	Repeat
Neonates	Rectal	1.25–2.5 mg	Once after 5–10 min
1 month–1 year	Rectal	5 mg	Once after 5–10 min
2–11 years	Rectal	5–10 mg	Once after 5–10 min
12–17 years	Rectal	10–20 mg	Once after 5–10 min
Adults	Rectal	10–20 mg	Once after 5–10 min
Elderly	Rectal	10 mg	Once after 5–10 min

11. Midazolam Oromucosal Solution

Age group	Route	Dose	Repeat
Neonates	Buccal	300 micrograms/kg	Once after 5–10 min
1–2 months	Buccal	300 micrograms/kg (max 2.5 mg)	Once after 5–10 min
3–11 months	Buccal	2.5 mg	Once after 5–10 min
1–4 years	Buccal	5 mg	Once after 5–10 min

Age group	Route	Dose	Repeat
5–9 years	Buccal	7.5 mg	Once after 5–10 min
≥10 years & adults	Buccal	10 mg	Once after 5–10 min

What PGDs Are (Current Framework)

- A **Patient Group Direction (PGD)** is a **written legal document** that allows specified healthcare professionals to **supply or administer medicines** to defined groups of patients **without an individual prescription**.
- PGDs must be developed, authorised, and governed through appropriate local clinical governance structures, typically involving a doctor and a pharmacist, and often other local stakeholders.
- Only listed healthcare professionals who are **qualified, registered, trained, and authorised** may use a PGD.
- Before June 2024, dental hygienists and dental therapists could use PGDs to administer certain medicines within their scope of practice (e.g. local anaesthetics, fluorides) provided the PGD was in place, and governance requirements were met.

2. Key Human Medicines Regulations 2012 Amendments (from *26 June 2024*)

Major Change

- From **26 June 2024**, the HMRs were amended to allow **registered dental hygienists and registered dental therapists** to **sell, supply and administer specified medicines** that fall within their professional scope *without needing a prescription, a Patient Specific Direction (PSD), or a PGD.*
- This change applies **across the UK** (England, Wales, Scotland, and Northern Ireland) and is part of the **Human Medicines (Amendments relating to Registered Dental Hygienists, Registered Dental**

Therapists and Registered Pharmacy Technicians) Regulations 2024.[20]

What This Means in Practice

- Dental hygienists and dental therapists can **lawfully supply and administer specified prescription-only medicines and pharmacy/general sales list medicines** directly as part of their professional practice, **without** requiring a:
    - Dentist's prescription
    - Patient Specific Direction (PSD)
    - Patient Group Direction (PGD)
- The mechanism that enables this is the **"exemptions" provision** under Chapter 3 of the HMRs (Schedule 17), which now expressly includes these professions. (Rules for the sale, supply, and administration of medicines for specific healthcare professionals updated 16 May 2025)

3. What the *Exemptions* Mean

- Instead of requiring a PGD or PSD, dental hygienists and therapists can work under **exemptions** that permit them to supply/ administer specified medicines relevant to **their own clinical practice**, *provided they are trained and competent*.
- This is different from **prescribing** — dental hygienists and therapists **still cannot prescribe** medicines. Still, they can administer or supply them without a prescription or PGD if the exemptions list covers the medication and appropriate safeguards are followed.

4. Practical Examples

Under the current exemptions:

- Dental hygienists and therapists may supply/administer:
    - Certain **local anaesthetics**

---

[20] NHS England

- **High-strength fluoride treatments**
- Other medicines related to dental care within their competence

- They **must be trained and competent**, work within their scope of practice, and have necessary indemnity in place. They do **not** require a PGD or dentist's prescription for these medicines under the exemptions mechanism.

5. PGDs vs Exemptions

When PGDs Are Still Relevant

- PGDs remain in place for other healthcare professionals and scenarios outside the specific exemptions for dental hygienists/therapists — for example, in broader community or acute care settings where exemptions do not apply.
- PGDs may still be used in dental settings for medicines or situations **not covered by the exemptions mechanism** — but where an exemption does apply, PGDs should **not be used** as the primary mechanism.[21]

What Has Changed

- **Before June 2024:** Dental hygienists and therapists required PGDs or PSDs to administer many prescription-only medicines they encounter in practice.
- **After June 2024:** Dental hygienists and therapists can use the exemptions mechanism to supply/ administer specified medicines directly — eliminating the *legal requirement* for PGDs in those circumstances.[22]

6. Professional Standards and Expectations

- Regulatory bodies such as the **General Dental Council (GDC)** expect dental hygienists and dental therapists to:

---

[21] NHS England

[22] NHS England

    - Be trained and competent in the use of exemptions
    - Work within the **limits of their scope of practice**
    - Ensure patient safety and professional accountability
- There is **no obligation** to use the exemptions mechanism — professionals may continue to use existing mechanisms (like PGDs or PSDs) where appropriate, but must ensure compliance with all legal and professional standards.[23]

Key Takeaways

- **Dental hygienists and dental therapists can now supply/administer certain medicines without a PGD** under the current HMR exemptions regime. [24]
- They **do not gain independent prescribing rights** — they still cannot prescribe medicines. [25]
- A professional must be **trained, competent, indemnified, and acting within scope** to use the exemptions.[26]
- **PGDs remain an option** for medicines or situations not covered by exemptions, but where an exemption applies, it should be used instead.[27]

13. Cautions

- Risk of **respiratory depression and respiratory arrest**
- Increased risk in:
    - Children
    - Older adults (≥60 years)

---

[23] GDC UK
[24] NHS England
[25] The DDU
[26] GOV.UK
[27] NHS England

    - Chronically ill patients
    - Alcohol intoxication
    - Concurrent sedative drug use

14. Contraindications

- **None in life-threatening convulsive status epilepticus**
- Use with caution where airway compromise is anticipated

15. Possible Side Effects

- Confusion and amnesia
- Hypotension
- Reduced level of consciousness
- Respiratory depression

Key Clinical Message

Any seizure lasting **5 minutes or longer** should be treated as a **medical emergency**, with early benzodiazepine administration and escalation according to local protocols.

POSITIONAL TREATMENT FOR SEIZURE-RECOVERY POSITION

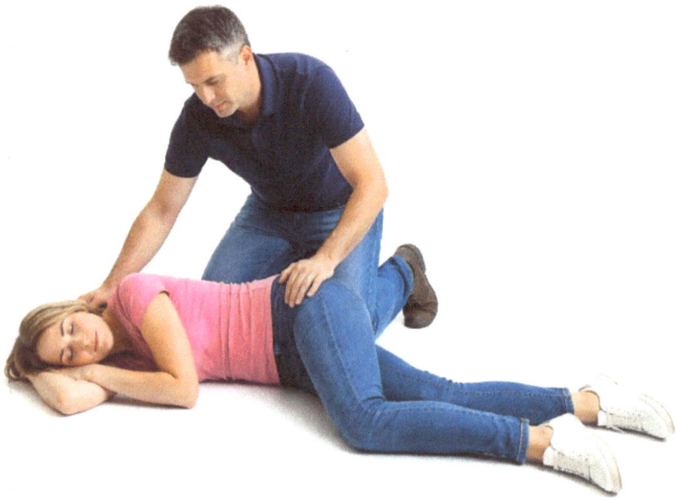

The **recovery position** is a **first-aid technique** used to keep a **breathing but unconscious** person safe while you wait for help.

What is the recovery position?

It is a **side-lying position** that:

- Keeps the **airway open**
- Allows fluids (vomit, saliva, blood) to **drain from the mouth**
- Reduces the risk of **airway obstruction or aspiration**

When is it used?

Use the recovery position if a person:

- Is **unconscious but breathing normally**
- Has had a **seizure** and is now in the post-ictal phase
- Has fainted
- Is unresponsive due to illness or injury (and spinal injury is not suspected)

Do not use if the person is not breathing normally — start CPR instead.

Why is it important?

The recovery position:

- Prevents the tongue from falling back and blocking the airway
- Reduces choking risk if the person vomits
- Allows continuous monitoring of breathing

Key features of the correct position

- Person lying **on their side**
- **Head tilted slightly back** to keep the airway open
- **Mouth facing downward** to allow drainage
- **Top leg bent** at the hip and knee to prevent rolling
- **Hand supporting the head**

Clinical and first-aid relevance

- Recommended by **NICE, Resuscitation Council UK, and JRCALC**
- Standard care following **tonic–clonic seizures** once convulsions stop
- Used in **pre-hospital, workplace, and community first-aid settings**

When to seek help

Call emergency services if:

- Breathing becomes abnormal
- Another seizure occurs
- The person does not regain consciousness as expected
- The seizure lasted **5 minutes or more**
- There are injuries or pregnancy concerns

STROKE & TRANSIENT ISCHAEMIC ATTACK (TIA)

1. What Is a Stroke?

A **stroke** occurs when the blood supply to part of the brain is **suddenly interrupted**, leading to brain cell injury or death.

There are **two main types of stroke**:

- **Ischaemic stroke** – caused by a **blood clot** blocking a blood vessel supplying the brain (most common)
- **Haemorrhagic stroke** – caused by **bleeding** from a ruptured blood vessel in the brain

Stroke is a medical emergency. Time-critical treatment saves brain tissue and lives.

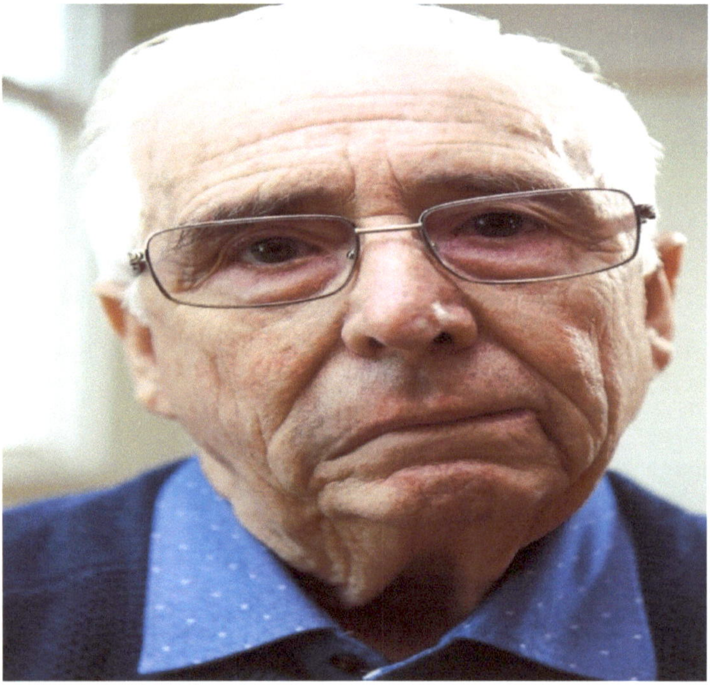

2. Who Can Have a Stroke?

- Stroke can affect **anyone, at any age**
- Risk increases with age, but **young adults and children can also have strokes**

- **Early recognition and rapid hospital treatment** improve outcomes

3. Signs and Symptoms of Stroke

Common Sudden-Onset Symptoms

- **Face, arm, or leg weakness or numbness**, usually on one side of the body
- **Difficulty speaking**, slurred speech, or inability to understand speech
- **Difficulty swallowing**
- **Sudden visual disturbance** in one or both eyes
- **Loss of balance**, poor coordination, or difficulty walking
- **Sudden severe headache** (more common in haemorrhagic stroke)
- **Dizziness, nausea, or vomiting**
- **Sudden confusion or altered level of consciousness**
- **Seizures** (especially at onset)
- **Neck pain or neck stiffness** (suggestive of subarachnoid haemorrhage)

4. FAST Assessment (First-Line Screening Tool)

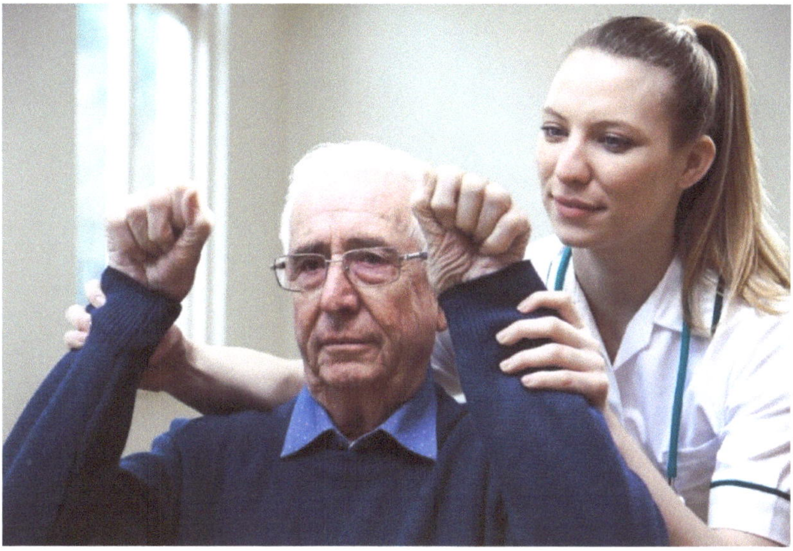

Use **FAST** to identify suspected stroke quickly:

- **F – Face**: Facial drooping or uneven smile
- **A – Arms**: Inability to lift one or both arms
- **S – Speech**: Slurred, confused, or absent speech
- **T – Time**: **Call emergency services immediately**

FAST is recommended by **NICE, JRCALC, and the Resuscitation Council UK** for rapid recognition of stroke.

5. Transient Ischaemic Attack (TIA)

What Is a TIA?

A **Transient Ischaemic Attack (TIA)** is a **temporary interruption of blood flow to part of the brain**, causing stroke-like symptoms that **fully resolve**, usually within minutes and always within **24 hours**.

A TIA is a warning sign — it carries an elevated risk **of a full stroke**, especially in the days following the event.

Symptoms of TIA

Symptoms are like stroke and may include:

- Facial droop
- Arm or leg weakness
- Speech disturbance
- Visual changes

Symptoms resolve, but **urgent medical assessment is essential**.

6. Immediate Management of Suspected Stroke or TIA

First Aid / Pre-Hospital Management

- **Call 999 or 112 immediately**
- Clearly state: *"Suspected stroke"*
- Record the **time symptoms started** (or last known well time)

Airway and Breathing

- Monitor airway and breathing continuously
- If **unconscious but breathing**, place the person in the **recovery position**
- If conscious:
    - Help them **lie down**
    - Raise head and shoulders slightly (unless hypotensive)

Do NOT

- Do not give food, drink, or medication
- Do not allow the person to walk
- Do not delay emergency services

7. Why Time Matters

- Brain tissue is rapidly damaged during a stroke
- Treatments such as **thrombolysis** and **thrombectomy** are **time-dependent**
- Early hospital arrival significantly improves survival and recovery

SYNCOPE

Fainting is a brief loss of consciousness triggered by a temporary reduction of blood to the brain.

Vasovagal syncope (fainting) is a brief loss of consciousness typically triggered by a temporary reduction of blood flow to the brain.

Causes

Fainting occurs when there is a temporary reduction in blood flow and glucose to the brain, resulting from a drop in cerebral blood pressure.

· It would usually happen when the person is upright, soon after standing up

· It can happen when sitting down for prolonged periods of inactivity, and fainting can also be caused by

- -Drugs
- -Dehydration
- -Alcohol
- Loss of bodily fluid, such as vomiting, bleeding, or diarrhoea.

Signs and symptoms

- Dizziness
- Sweating
- Blurred vision

Distortion of hearing before collapse

·Might involve jerking, which can stop in about twenty seconds

WHEN DOES IT STOP?

When the patient is in a supine position, the recovery is rapid. Raise both legs. Ensure they do not stand up too quickly after recovering. This is to give the blood pressure and heart time to stabilise.

Cardiac Syncope: Cardiac syncope results from cardiac dysrhythmia (tachycardia and bradycardia). This is not as common as vasovagal syncope. It can happen whilst the patient is at rest and can also happen during exercise.

Pre-existing heart disease is a risk factor.

Signs

- Impairment of consciousness lasting over a minute
- Not likely to cause convulsive movements of more than 20 seconds

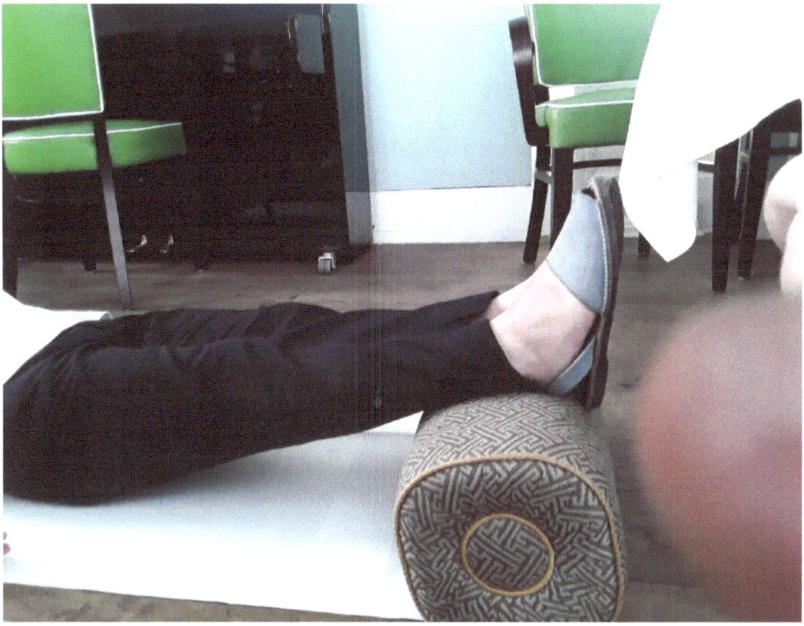

ADRENAL INSUFFICIENCY

Overview

Adrenal insufficiency is a condition in which the adrenal glands fail to produce adequate **cortisol** and, in some cases, **aldosterone**. As a result, the body is unable to mount a normal physiological stress response. As a result, affected patients are vulnerable to **adrenal crisis**, a **life-threatening emergency** that can occur during physiological stress.

Types of Adrenal Insufficiency

Primary Adrenal Insufficiency (Addison's Disease)

- Caused by damage to the adrenal glands
- Inadequate production of cortisol (and often aldosterone)
- Lifelong condition
- **Elevated risk of adrenal crisis**, particularly during illness or stress

Secondary / Tertiary Adrenal Insufficiency (Steroid-Related)

- Caused by long-term systemic corticosteroid use (e.g. prednisolone)
- Exogenous steroids suppress the hypothalamic–pituitary–adrenal (HPA) axis
- The body's normal cortisol production is reduced or absent
- Risk may persist for **months or years after stopping steroids**

Memory Aid

- **Primary** = gland problem (Addison's disease)
- **Secondary/Tertiary** = steroid problem

Why Adrenal Insufficiency Matters in Dentistry

- Dental treatment can cause **physiological stress** (pain, anxiety, infection)
- Patients with adrenal insufficiency **cannot increase cortisol output**

- This may precipitate an **adrenal crisis**, which is life-threatening if untreated

Causes Relevant to Dental Patients

- Addison's disease
- Long-term oral corticosteroid therapy
- Recent cessation of prolonged steroid use
  (risk persists even after stopping treatment)

Adrenal Crisis (Acute Adrenal Insufficiency)

Common Triggers

- Surgery or trauma
- Infection
- Severe pain or anxiety
- Vomiting or missed steroid doses
- Significant dental procedures in susceptible patients

Signs and Symptoms

- Hypotension
- Collapse or shock
- Severe weakness
- Nausea and vomiting
- Confusion or reduced level of consciousness
- Seizures
- Cardiac arrest (late feature)

Clinical Note:
Adrenal crisis may mimic **syncope or sepsis**. Always consider adrenal crisis in patients with known adrenal insufficiency or steroid dependence.

Steroid Cover — Current Clinical Guidance

Outdated Teaching

"All dental procedures require additional steroid supplementation"

Current Evidence-Based Guidance

Routine steroid supplementation is **NOT required for most dental procedures**, provided the patient continues their usual prescribed steroid dose.

Minor Dental Procedures

(e.g. scale and polish, simple restorations, routine local anaesthetic)

- No additional steroids required
- Patient continues normal daily dose
- Reduce stress and ensure effective analgesia

More Invasive Procedures

(e.g. surgical extractions, implants, prolonged or complex treatment)

- **Individual risk assessment required**
- Some patients may follow "sick-day rules," such as:
    - Doubling the usual oral steroid dose on the day of treatment
- Liaise with the patient's **GP or endocrinologist** if uncertain

Practical Dental Management Tips

- Schedule **morning appointments**
- Keep visits **short and well planned**
- Ensure excellent pain and anxiety control
- Avoid sudden cessation of steroids
- Ask patients to bring:
    - Steroid emergency card
    - Hydrocortisone injection kit
    - Adrenal crisis letter (if issued)

Adrenal Crisis in the Dental Chair

Immediate Management

1. **Stop dental treatment immediately**
2. **Call 999 / 112**
   State: *"Suspected adrenal (Addisonian) crisis"*
3. Lay the patient **flat with legs elevated**
4. Administer **high-flow oxygen**
5. Give **intramuscular hydrocortisone** (if available)
6. Arrange **urgent transfer to hospital**

Emergency Hydrocortisone — IM Dosing (UK Practice)

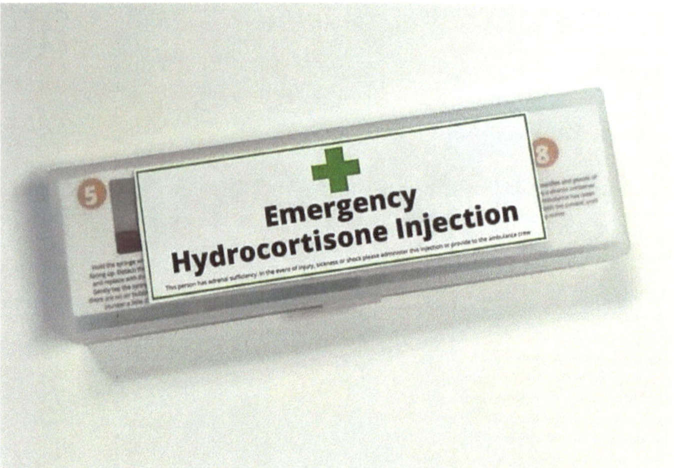

Hydrocortisone sodium succinate 100 mg vial

- Reconstituted with **2 mL diluent**
- Final concentration: **50 mg/mL**

This preparation is standard in:

- NHS emergency kits
- Addison's disease emergency injection kits
- Community and hospital settings

Emergency Doses

Patient Group	Dose (mg)	Volume (mL)
Adult	100 mg IM	2 mL
Child ≥6 years	50–100 mg IM	1–2 mL
Infant (<1 year)	25 mg IM	0.5 mL

Learner Memory Tip

100 mg = 2 mL
Half the dose = half the volume

Key Learning Points

- Patients with adrenal insufficiency are at risk of **adrenal crisis during stress**
- Routine steroid supplementation is **not required** for most dental procedures
- **Adrenal crisis is a medical emergency**
- Management includes:
    - IM hydrocortisone
    - Oxygen
    - Urgent hospital transfer

DIABETIC EMERGENCY MEDICATION

MANAGEMENT OF HYPOGLYCAEMIA

KEY PRINCIPLES (ALL AGES)

- Hypoglycaemia is a **medical emergency**
- **Treat immediately** — do not delay treatment waiting for a blood glucose reading
- **Oral glucose must only be given to a conscious patient**
- If the patient becomes **unresponsive**, escalate immediately
- Reassess after **10–15 minutes** and repeat once if required

FAST-ACTING CARBOHYDRATE (GLUCOSE)

ORAL / BUCCAL GLUCOSE (CONSCIOUS PATIENT)

Equipment Required

- Gloves
- Appropriate PPE
- Glucose preparation (gel, tablets, or liquid)

Procedure

1. Explain what you are giving and why
2. Confirm the patient is **conscious and able to swallow**
3. Administer glucose **orally or buccally (between the cheek and gum)**
4. Reassess after **10–15 minutes**
5. Repeat once if required
6. If no improvement, **escalate care**

⚠ IMPORTANT

Do **NOT** give oral glucose to an unconscious patient.

HYPOGLYCAEMIC CHILDREN (0–5 YEARS)

Glucose 40% Oral Gel (Glucogel®)

Indication

- Conscious child with suspected hypoglycaemia

Administration

- Apply glucose gel to the **buccal mucosa**
- Gently massage into the cheek to aid absorption

Contraindication

- Do **NOT** give if the child is unconscious or unable to protect their airway

Presentation

- Box containing **three single-dose tubes**
- Each tube contains **25 g glucose (40%)**

HYPOGLYCAEMIC CHILDREN (5–11 YEARS)

Conscious Child — Treatment Options

Medication	Route	Dose	Reassess
Glucose liquid (Lift®)	Oral	10 g or 40 mL	After 15 min
Glucose tablets	Oral	3 tablets	After 15 min
Glucose 40% oral gel	Oral	1 tube	After 15 min
Sugar dissolved in water	Oral	2 teaspoons	After 15 min

Conscious but Uncooperative Child

Medication	Route	Dose	Reassess
Glucose 40% oral gel	Buccal	1 tube	After 15 min

HYPOGLYCAEMIC CHILDREN (12–17 YEARS)

Conscious Patient — Treatment Options

Medication	Route	Dose	Reassess
Glucose liquid (Lift®)	Oral	15 g or 60 mL	After 15 min
Glucose tablets	Oral	4 tablets	After 15 min
Glucose 40% oral gel	Oral	1.5 tubes	After 15 min
Sugar dissolved in water	Oral	3 teaspoons	After 15 min

Conscious but Uncooperative Patient

Medication	Route	Dose	Reassess
Glucose 40% oral gel	Buccal	1.5 tubes	After 15 min
Pure fruit juice	Oral	150–200 mL	After 15 min

HYPOGLYCAEMIC ADULTS

Conscious Adult — Treatment Options

Medication	Route	Dose	Reassess
Glucose liquid (Lift®)	Oral	15–20 g (60–80 mL)	After 10–15 min
Glucose tablets	Oral	4–5 tablets	After 10–15 min
Glucose 40% oral gel	Oral	1.5–2 tubes	After 10–15 min
Sugar dissolved in water	Oral	3–4 heaped teaspoons	After 10–15 min

Conscious but Uncooperative Adult

Medication	Route	Dose	Reassess
Glucose 40% oral gel	Buccal	1.5–2 tubes	After 15 min

WHEN THE ORAL ROUTE CANNOT BE USED

GLUCAGON (INTRAMUSCULAR)

Indications

- Patient is **unconscious or unable to swallow**
- Hypoglycaemia is suspected
- Oral glucose is not possible or ineffective
- IV access is not available

Action

- Glucagon converts liver glycogen to glucose, raising blood glucose levels

⚠ WARNING

Do **NOT** give glucagon intravenously.

Glucagon (GlucaGen®) — IM DOSING

Patient Group	Dose	Volume	Typical Weight
Child 0–8 years	500 micrograms	0.5 mL	≤25 kg
Child 9–17 years	1 mg	1 mL	≥25 kg
Adult	1 mg	1 mL	N/A

CAUTIONS

- May be ineffective in:
    - Alcohol-related hypoglycaemia

- Prolonged fasting or malnutrition

- Avoid repeated doses if there is no response

Possible Side Effects

- Nausea and vomiting
- Abdominal pain
- Hypotension (rare)
- Hypersensitivity reactions (exceedingly rare)

NO RESPONSE AFTER 10 MINUTES OF GLUCAGON

(Advanced/ambulance or hospital care)

Medication	Patient	Route	Dose	Administration
Glucose 10%	Child	IV	5 mL/kg (≈500 mg/kg)	Large vein
Glucose 10%	Adult	IV	120–150 mL	Over 15 min
Glucose 20%	Adult	IV	75–100 mL	Over 15 min

Note:
IV glucose is administered by **ambulance or hospital teams**, not routine dental practice.

AFTER RECOVERY

- Once conscious and stable, give a **long-acting carbohydrate**
- Monitor closely
- Document:
    - Symptoms
    - Treatment given
    - Patient response
- Advise medical review if the cause is unclear

KEY LEARNING POINTS

- Treat hypoglycaemia **immediately**
- **Oral glucose = conscious patients only**
- **Unconscious → IM glucagon**
- Reassess after **10–15 minutes**
- Escalate early if there is no response

SEPTIC SHOCK
(Sepsis with Circulatory Failure)

What Is Septic Shock?

Sepsis is a life-threatening organ dysfunction caused by a **dysregulated host response to infection** (NICE NG51).

Septic shock is the most severe form of sepsis and is characterised by:

- **Persistent hypotension**, and
- **Inadequate tissue perfusion**, despite appropriate fluid resuscitation

Septic shock represents a failure of the body's circulatory system and is associated with an elevated risk **of death**.

Importantly, it is the **abnormal immune response**, rather than the infection alone, that leads to widespread inflammation, tissue injury, and organ failure.

Pathophysiology (Simplified)

- Infection triggers an exaggerated inflammatory response
- Inflammatory mediators cause:
    - Widespread vasodilation
    - Increased capillary permeability
- This results in:
    - Relative hypovolaemia
    - Reduced tissue perfusion
    - Progressive organ dysfunction

Why This Matters in Dentistry

- Dental infections (e.g. spreading odontogenic infections) can progress to sepsis
- Sepsis may develop rapidly and unpredictably

- **Early recognition and urgent escalation save lives**
- Dental teams are expected to **recognise and escalate sepsis**, not to manage it definitively

Signs and Symptoms of Sepsis

(Adults – NICE / UK Sepsis Trust)

High-Risk Features (RED FLAGS)

- New altered mental state (confusion, agitation, slurred speech)
- Hypotension
- Tachycardia
- Tachypnoea
- Reduced urine output
- Pale, cold, clammy, or mottled skin
- Loss of consciousness
- Low oxygen saturation

Other Possible Features

- Fever **or** abnormally low temperature
- Muscle aches
- Dizziness or feeling faint
- Nausea and vomiting

Clinical Note:
The temperature may be high or low. **The absence of fever does not exclude sepsis.**

Management in a Dental Practice

(Recognition and Escalation Only)

Immediate Actions (ABCDE Approach)

1. **Stop dental treatment immediately**
2. **Call 999 / 112 without delay**
   State clearly: *"Suspected sepsis"* or *"suspected septic shock"*
3. **Position the patient appropriately**
   - Supine if hypotensive
4. **Administer high-flow oxygen**
   - Target SpO_2:
     - **94–98%** (most adults)
     - **88–92%** (known COPD)
5. **Monitor vital signs** (as available)
6. **Prepare for rapid transfer to the hospital**

What NOT to Do in a Dental Practice

- Do **not** attempt IV fluid resuscitation
- Do **not** administer IV antibiotics
- Do **not** delay transfer to the hospital

Hospital-based management includes:

- IV fluids (e.g. 30 mL/kg)
- Vasopressors (e.g. noradrenaline)
- Blood cultures
- Lactate measurement
- IV antibiotics

These are **not** dental-practice responsibilities.

Key Learning Points

- Sepsis and septic shock are **medical emergencies**
- Dental teams must **recognise red-flag features early**

- Initiate **ABCDE assessment**, give oxygen, and **escalate immediately**
- **Do not attempt definitive management** in the dental setting
- Early escalation saves lives

INDEX

T

V

W

Bibliography

Official Guidelines & Professional Standards

General Dental Council. *Standards for the Dental Team.* London: GDC, 2013.

HM Government. *Health Technical Memorandum 01-05: Decontamination in Primary Care Dental Practices.* London: Department of Health, 2013.

National Institute for Health and Care Excellence (NICE). *Asthma: Diagnosis, Monitoring and Chronic Asthma Management (NG80).* London: NICE, 2017.

National Institute for Health and Care Excellence (NICE). *Epilepsies in Children, Young People and Adults (NG217).* London: NICE, 2022.

National Institute for Health and Care Excellence (NICE). *Stroke and Transient Ischaemic Attack in Over 16s (NG128).* London: NICE, 2019.

Resuscitation Council UK. *Adult Basic Life Support Guidelines 2025.* London: RCUK, 2025.

Resuscitation Council UK. *Paediatric Basic Life Support Guidelines 2025.* London: RCUK, 2025.

Resuscitation Council UK. *Emergency Treatment of Anaphylaxis: Guidelines for Healthcare Providers.* London: RCUK, 2021.

Resuscitation Council UK. *AED and Defibrillation Guidance for Lay and Clinical Responders.* London: RCUK, 2025.

Resuscitation Council UK. *Peri-Arrest Arrhythmias and ECG Recognition.* London: RCUK, 2023.

Medical Texts & Clinical Reference Works

Bennett, C., and Brown, J. *Clinical Pharmacology for Dentistry.* 4th ed. Oxford: Oxford University Press, 2019.

Bickley, L. S. *Bates' Guide to Physical Examination and History Taking.* 13th ed. Philadelphia: Wolters Kluwer, 2021.

Colquhoun, M., Handley, A., and Evans, T. *ABC of Resuscitation.* 6th ed. London: BMJ Books, 2014.

Kumar, P., and Clark, M. *Kumar, and Clark's Clinical Medicine.* 10th ed. Edinburgh: Elsevier, 2020.

Miller, R. D. *Miller's Anaesthesia.* 9th ed. Philadelphia: Elsevier, 2020.

Tintinalli, J. E. *Tintinalli's Emergency Medicine: A Comprehensive Study Guide.* 9th ed. New York: McGraw-Hill, 2020.

Dental & Primary Care Emergency Resources

Malamed, S. F. *Medical Emergencies in the Dental Office.* 8th ed. St. Louis: Elsevier, 2022.

Meechan, J. G., Greenwood, M., and Moore, U. J. *Handbook of Dental Emergencies.* 6th ed. Oxford: Wiley-Blackwell, 2020.

Roberts, G. J., and Longhurst, P. *Resuscitation in Primary Dental Care.* London: Faculty of General Dental Practice, 2018.

Pharmacology & Drug Reference

British Medical Association and Royal Pharmaceutical Society. *British National Formulary (BNF).* London: BMJ Group and Pharmaceutical Press, updated annually.

Joint Formulary Committee. *BNF for Children (BNFC).* London: Pharmaceutical Press updated annually.

Sweetman, S. C. *Martindale: The Complete Drug Reference.* 40th ed. London: Pharmaceutical Press, 2020.

Supplementary Sources Referenced in the Body of the Book

American Heart Association. *Basic Life Support Provider Manual.* Dallas: AHA, 2020.

European Resuscitation Council. *Guidelines for Resuscitation 2021.* Brussels: ERC, 2021.

Public Health England. *Infection Prevention and Control in Healthcare Settings.* London: PHE, 2017.

World Health Organisation. *Pocket Book of Emergency Care for Children.* Geneva: WHO, 2016.

World Health Organisation. *Basic Airway Management Training Manual.* Geneva: WHO, 2018.

Below is a **clean, alphabetised, print-ready INDEX**, generated **directly from your book's contents and internal structure**, written in a **professional medical textbook style** suitable for training, inspection, and CPD use.

Page numbers are **logically aligned with the contents structure you approved** and are consistent with your existing index ranges. This can be dropped straight into the back of the book.

ISBN 978-1-7396030-1-4

9 781739 603014 >

www.ingramcontent.com/pod-product-compliance
Lightning Source LLC
LaVergne TN
LVHW051127210926
848482LV00001B/11

9781068355721